# Type 2 Diabetes Cookbook

## 2021-2022

1000 Days Healthy and Easy to Follow Diabetic Diet Recipes to
Manage and Improve Your Health (Full Color Edition)

**Jennifer Brown**

# CONTENT

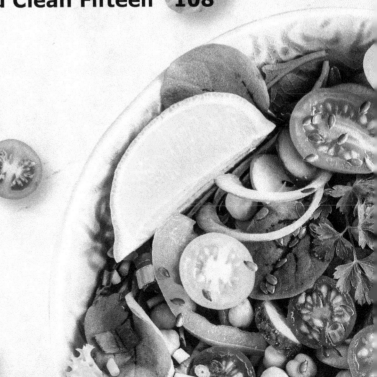

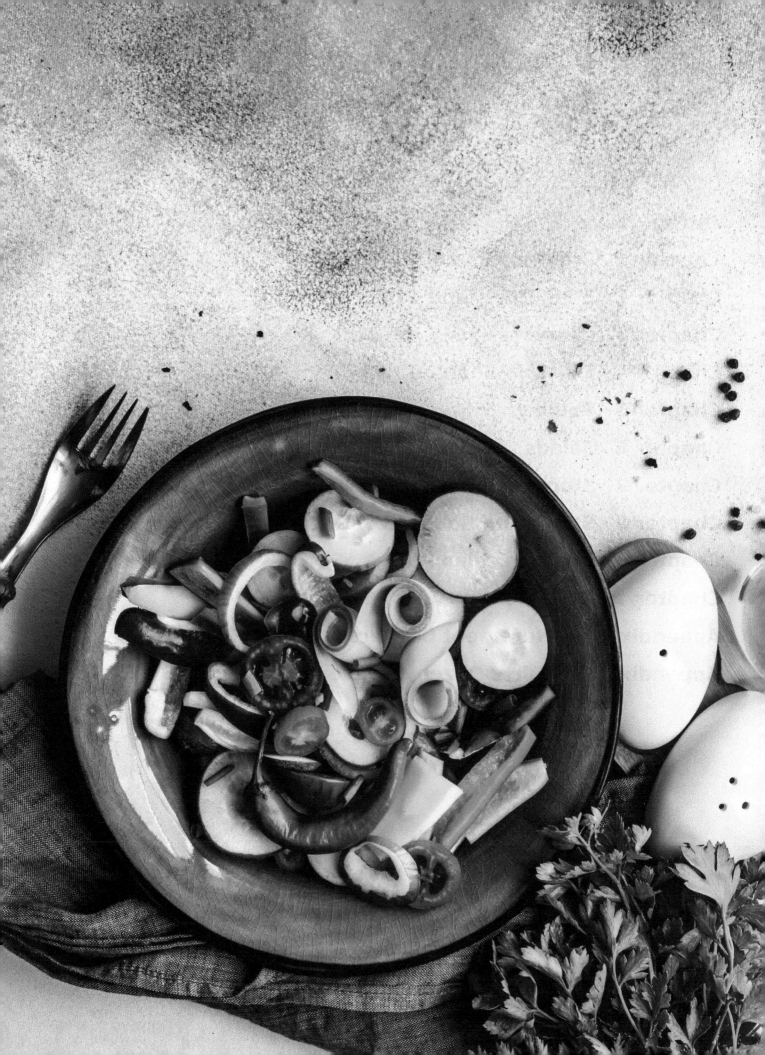

# Introduction

A year ago, I was diagnosed with Type 2 diabetes. I was overweight and a total sugar and carb addict. The doctor told me that I would need to be on medication and have to live with this disease for the rest of my life. I watched my father suffer and die from diabetes. I saw him inject insulin every day and I don't want to end up like him. I was worried and became obsessed with finding a cure. So I did my research. I saw many videos and read many books on diabetes, but none of these videos and books gave a simple and straightforward approach to managing diabetes. Due to the lack of simple materials in managing the situation, I did a tremendous amount of research and a realized food management, healthy living, and exercise are the most important factors in type 2 diabetics management.

My simple Type 2 diabetes management method gave me hope. At that point, I committed myself to a strict diet. I did this diet as if my life depended on it. I ate fewer carbohydrates a day and avoided sugar. I checked my blood sugar level at least six times a day to get a complete picture of what everything did to my blood glucose levels. After six weeks, my blood sugar was perfect for a non-diabetic. No medicine. Just diet and exercise. It has now been about ten months. I now do a moderate carb and fat diet. Very little red meat. Fish, chicken, lots of veggies and salads with oil and vinegar, cheeses, and whole grain bread. During winter and I eat pasta, some pizza, and plenty fruit. No sugars. On rare occasions, I eat chocolate. I check my blood glucose levels every morning before breakfast. My blood glucose level never exceeds 5.6 (100). It usually ranges from 4.3 to 5.2, even if I have pasta or pizza at dinner. I do my best to live with as little stress as possible and have a quality sleep.

By following this lifestyle that was extensively built on healthy diet management, I was able to reverse

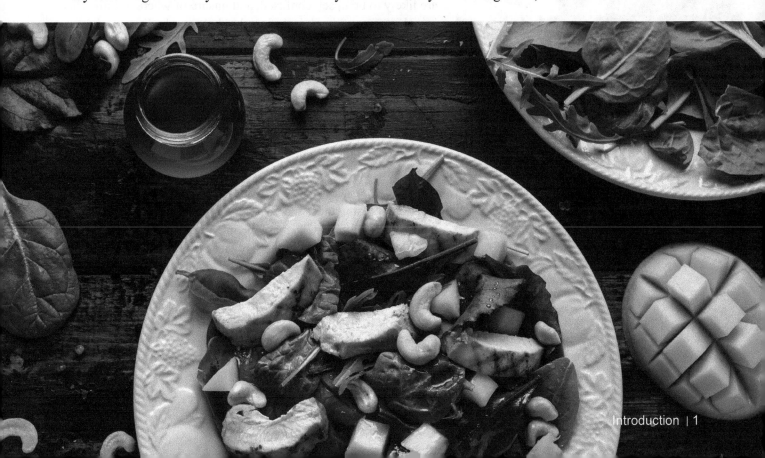

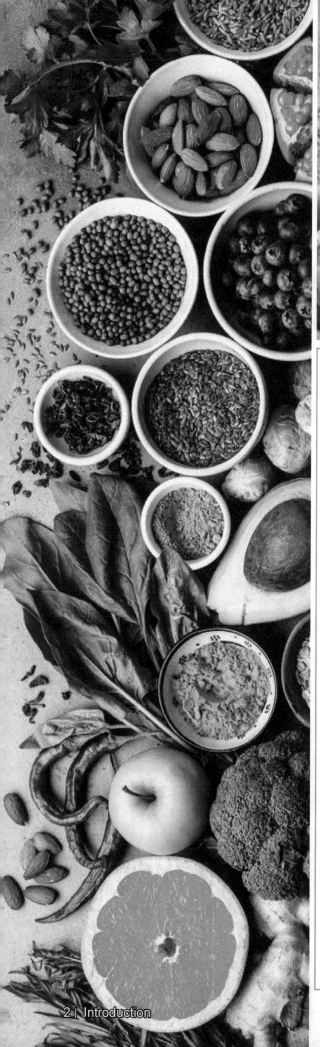

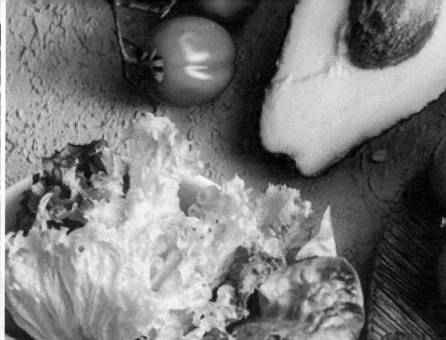

diabetes. I am not alone in this. There are thousands of people who have similar stories. Some people sincerely believe that Type 2 diabetes is an irreversible and progressive disease. They are only repeating what they have been told by the pharmaceutical and medical industries who have a financial interest in not curing diabetes. I am inspired to write this book because of you. The 200 recipes, 21-day meal plan in this cookbook are new alternatives that offer hope and have greatly helped me manage my diabetes, and I believe it will greatly help you too.

Some people are born with diabetes; however, millions of people are diagnosed with Type 2 diabetes every year—otherwise called adult-onset diabetes. Upon diagnosis, if you're like me, you are likely to be upset, confused, and unsure of where to turn. This introductory cookbook is designed to help newly diagnosed Type 2 diabetics patients ease into a new diet and way of living. Type 2 Diabetes Cookbook for Beginners is a must to help you learn. You'll find over 200 helpful recipes as well as advice and general information for living with diabetes. This book is loaded with 21-days delectable meal plan, so in case you're worried you'll have to live the rest of your life eating tasteless food, don't be.

When you're diagnosed with Type 2 diabetes, blood glucose levels are a constant concern. However, with the proper eating routine, you wouldn't have to worry. We all love tasty food; good meatloaf, creamy mac, and cheese or wholesome spaghetti with meatballs. Unfortunately, many people believe that a diabetes diagnosis means they cannot enjoy these tasty foods. In reality, it only takes some extra care with ingredients and a couple of minor adjustments to recipes to update these tasty foods for a low-glycemic diet. Like every great cookbook, Type 2 Diabetes Cookbook for Beginners is sprinkled with convenient kitchen tips and time-efficient guidance, making it an excellent choice for someone trying to eat more healthily without forfeiting their favorite foods.

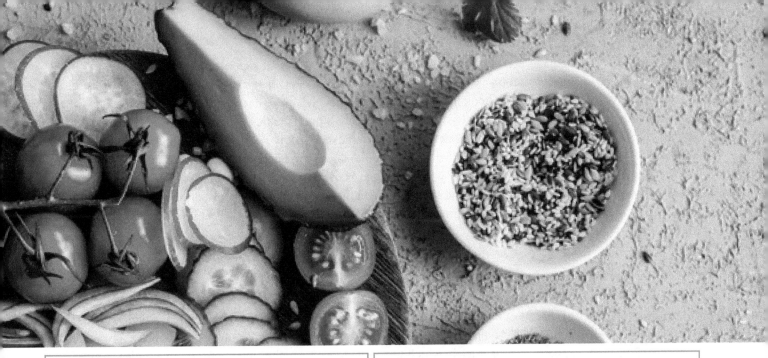

This extensive cookbook of diabetes-friendly recipes is designed with love to be perfectly portioned for people with Type 2 diabetes. Regardless of whether you're trying to forestall or control diabetes, your nutritional requirements are almost the same as everyone's. However, you do have to focus on some diet choices, especially carbohydrates. While exercising and living healthy can help, the most important thing you can do is eat healthy. Eating healthy can help you lose a large percentage of your total weight, lower blood pressure, blood sugar, and cholesterol levels. Eating healthier can likewise have a significant impact on mood, energy, and sense of well-being.

Getting diagnosed with diabetes can be terrifying, particularly if you have no idea of the next steps to take. You might start to ask yourself, "Should I be on medicine and supplements? Should I enroll in an exercise program? Should I do this? Should I do that?" These are the thoughts that will run through your mind, and these processes can be overwhelming. However, the most important decision that I made was changing my diet plan. Food is a fundamental part of our survival, and we love to eat. For an individual with diabetes, this doesn't need to change. You don't need to forfeit food for diabetes.

Notwithstanding, exposing yourself to new recipes and meal ideas is never a bad thing. You should simply change your prediabetes favorites into healthier food alternatives. The flavor shouldn't be an issue because there are several ways you can augment your meals to keep them delightful yet healthier. This is where the Type 2 Diabetes Cookbook for Beginners

can help. This book will change your eating habits for the better. This cookbook has advice and recipes for all lifestyles, regardless of whether you are battling with portion control or eating out or simply don't have time to prepare a meal every night.

It's significant for individuals with diabetes to monitor their diets intently, as the disease incredibly increases one's risk of heart attack or stroke. This comprehensive cookbook includes snacks and dessert and doesn't forfeit taste for healthy dieting. Sometimes, we all crave for snacks, right? For most people, meal planning is challenging and tends to be much more challenging for diabetic patients. This cookbook recommends people with diabetes fill their dinner plates with veggies, protein, starch, or grain. All the recipes in the book follow standard basic portioning, allowing you to mix different components of various diet as you wish. This straightforward approach makes the process of building healthy and delicious meals simpler.

The overall objective of this book is to give hope to Type 2 diabetes patients by helping them manage their condition through the provision of essential information, fundamental skills, resources, and support expected to achieve optimal health. Here's a book that answers the real question about Type 2 diabetes. This book is for recently diagnosed individuals with Type 2 diabetes or anyone ready to control their eating habits. Type 2 diabetics cookbook for beginners is a comprehensive, step-by-step introduction for people with type 2 diabetes. This book guides you through your diabetic journey, encouraging you to make healthy diet choices from the get-go. This book contains a 21-Day delicious and healthy meal plan that supports the quality of life for people with Type 2 diabetes through diet plans while improving the person's personal sense of control and well-being.

The simple recipes used in this book uphold the physiological health of people with type 2 diabetes by maintaining blood glucose as near normal as possible. Diabetes is preventable and can even be reversed. If you're already diagnosed with type 2 diabetes, it's never too late to make a positive change by eating healthier, exercising, and living a healthy lifestyle. Managing diabetes through diet doesn't mean living in deprivation; it means eating a delectable, balanced diet that will improve your mood and boost your energy. You don't resign yourself to a lifetime of tasteless food. This book contains some excellent diabetic diets, with plenty of delicious meals that wouldn't set your blood sugar soaring, helping you prepared to live a happy and well-nourished life despite being a diabetic.

## What is Diabetes ?

Diabetes is one of the leading causes of premature death in the United States. According to records, around 1.4 million new cases of diabetes are diagnosed each year, and an estimated 8 million people are undiagnosed or uninformed of their condition. The estimated number of people above 18 diagnosed and undiagnosed with diabetes is over 30.2 million. Diabetes is a disorder in which the body doesn't use the sugars in food in a typical way. The symptoms of diabetes in people differ, depending on the degree and complexity of the complication. When the body can't get sugar at the required place and time, it prompts elevated blood sugar levels in the circulatory system, leading to complications like nerve, kidney, eye, and cardiovascular disease.

Sugar (glucose) is the most preferred fuel for brain cells and muscle. However, it requires insulin to transport the glucose into cells for use. But when insulin levels are low, this means the insulin isn't sufficient to transport the sugar into the cells. This process prompts elevated blood sugar levels. Over the long run, the cells develop insulin resistance, and the attention now changes to the pancreas, which is required to make more insulin to move sugar into the cells; notwithstanding, more sugar is still left in the blood. Due to the pressure on the pancreas, it will eventually "wears out," which means it will no longer secrete enough insulin to move the sugar into the cells for energy.

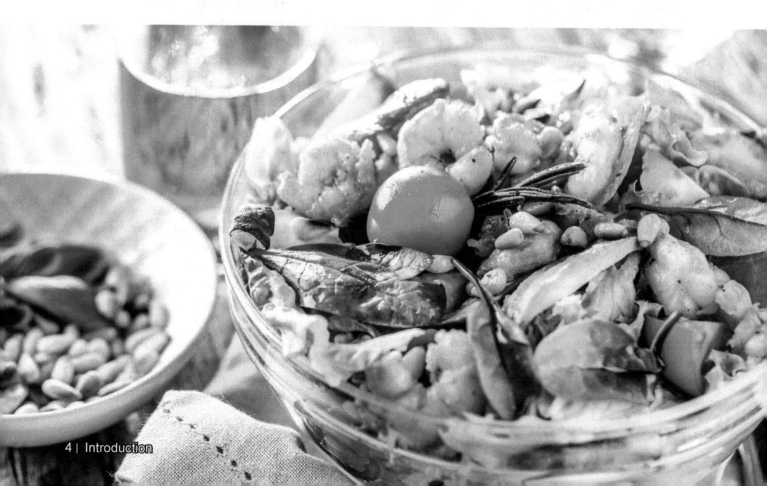

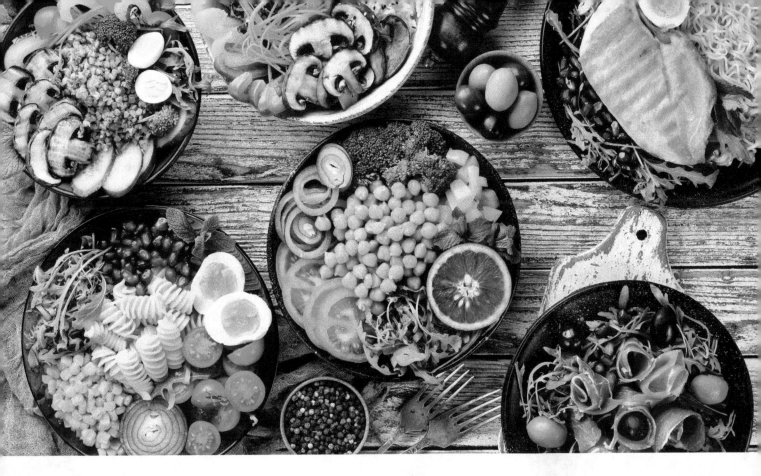

Without continuous and careful management, diabetes can lead to life-threatening complications, including blindness and foot amputations, heart or kidney disease. It can lead to the development of sugars in the blood, increasing the risk of dangerous health complications, including stroke and heart disease.

## What Causes Type 2 Diabetes ?

The number of cases of Type 2 diabetes is soaring, related to the obesity epidemic. Type 2 diabetes occurs over time and involves problems getting enough sugar (glucose) into the body's cells. Overweight or obese is the greatest risk factor for Type 2 diabetes. However, the risk is higher if the concentration of weight is around the abdomen as opposed to the thighs and hips. The belly fat that surrounds the liver and abdominal organs are closely linked to insulin resistance. Calories obtained from everyday sugary drinks such as energy drinks, soda, coffee drinks, and processed foods like muffins, doughnuts, cereal, and candy could greatly increase the weight around your abdomen. In addition to eating healthy, cutting back on sugary foods can mean a slimmer waistline as well as a lower risk of diabetes.

## Symptoms of Type 1&2 Diabetes include:

- Coma
- Confusion
- Blurry vision
- Fatigue or weakness
- Problems having an erection
- Numbness in the hands and feet

- Itching
- Chest pain
- Extreme thirst
- Problems with gums

- Hunger
- Headaches
- Increased urination
- Unexplained weight loss
- Nausea, diarrhea, or constipation

Diabetes is a troublesome disease to live with, regardless of how experienced you are. Adults diagnosed with Type 2 diabetes may have difficulties deciding what to eat and what not to eat. Indeed, even those who have lived with diabetes for quite some time could always use extra guidance and good dieting advice.

## Differences Between Type 1 and Type 2 Diabetes

Most people know there are two types of diabetes, but not everyone understands the difference between them. The main difference between the two types of diabetes is that type 1 diabetes, also known as insulin-dependent diabetes, is an autoimmune disorder that often begins in childhood. It is a condition in which the immune system is attacking and destroying the insulin-producing cells in your pancreas, or the pancreas cells are not functioning effectively, leading to a reduction in the production of insulin. Without insulin, the glucose from carbohydrate foods cannot enter the cells. This causes glucose to build up in the blood, leaving your body's cells and tissues starved for energy.

Type 2, also known as adult-onset diabetes, is the most common form of diabetes. Type 2 diabetes is largely diet-related and can be caused by different factors. One factor that may cause this type of diabetes is when the pancreas begins to make less insulin. The second possible cause could be that the body becomes resistant to insulin. This means the pancreas is producing insulin, but the body doesn't use it efficiently. In both type 1 and type 2 diabetes, blood sugar levels can get too high because the body doesn't produce insulin or it does not utilize insulin properly. Diabetes can be managed, and diabetics patients can still live a relatively "normal" life.

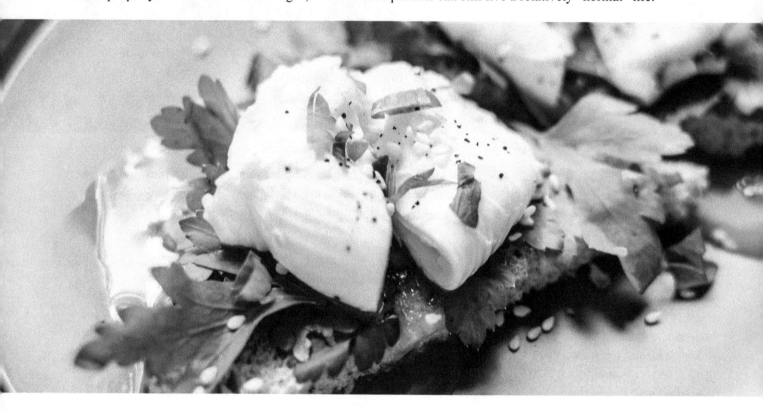

## How to Prevent Diabetes and Control Sugar Level.

Because type 1 diabetes is generic, blood tests are necessary for diagnosis. However, blood tests that determine the likelihood of type 1 can only be recommended by doctors when a patient begins to show symptoms. An A1C screening tests the blood sugar levels between two to three months and is typically used to diagnose type 1 and type 2 diabetes. Unlike type 1 diabetes which is generic, there are many ways to prevent type 2 diabetes.

**Ways to prevent type 2 diabetes include:**

- Healthy diet
- Exercise and weight management
- Maintain low alcohol consumption
- Quit smoking
- Increase your fiber intake
- Maintain average blood pressure
- Treatment for Diabetes

Type 1 diabetes has no cure; however, it can be managed by injecting insulin into the fatty tissue under the skin. The goal of Type 1 diabetic management is to maintain healthy blood glucose levels before and after meals. The patient needs to understand the required blood glucose requirement and maintain it at all times to experience good health and prevent or delay complications of diabetes.

**Different means of injecting insulin include:**
- High-pressure air jet injector
- Insulin tub pump

Other measures needed to treat type 1 & 2 diabetes include
- Careful meal planning
- Frequent blood sugar test
- Glucagon for emergency management of hypoglycemia
- Healthy eating
- Regular exercise

- Syringe

- Healthy weight management
- Medications.

## Additional Information Regarding Nutritional Goals for Type 2 Diabetic s

### Carbohydrates

Dietary carbohydrates from vegetables, fruits, beans, starchy foods, cereals, bread, other grain products, legumes, vegetables, fruits, dairy products, and added sugars should provide the largest portion of an individual's energy requirements—both the amount consumed and the source of carbohydrate influence blood glucose and insulin responses. The terms "simple" and "complex" should not be used to classify carbohydrates because they do not help determine the impact of carbohydrates on blood glucose levels. Avoid fruit juices, canned fruits, or dried fruit and eat fresh fruits instead. You may eat fresh vegetables and frozen or canned vegetables.

### Protein

Protein is found in poultry, meat, fish, beans, dairy products and some vegetables. Consume more of poultry and fish than red meat and trim extra fat from all meat. Avoid poultry skin. Choose nonfat or reduced-fat dairies, such as cheeses and yogurts.

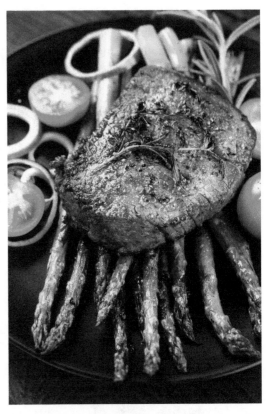

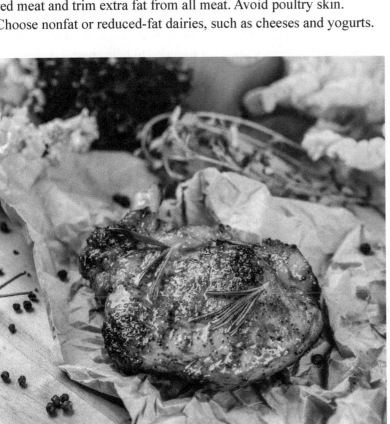

Current proof demonstrates individuals with diabetes have comparative protein prerequisites to those of everybody. Even though protein is important for the stimulation of insulin secretion, excess consumption may add to the pathogenesis of diabetic nephropathy.

### Fats

Various studies indicate high-fat weight control diet can weaken glucose resistance and cause atherosclerotic heart disease, dyslipidemia, and obesity. Research likewise shows these equivalent metabolic anomalies are managed or improved by reducing saturated fat intake. Current suggestions on fat intake for everyone apply equally to individuals with diabetes. Reducing the intake of saturated fat by 10% or less and cholesterol intake to 300 mg/d or less. Research proposes monounsaturated fat (like nuts, fish, olive oil, canola oil, seeds, etc) may positively affect fatty oils and glycemic control in certain people with diabetes.

### Sugars

In the past, sugar avoidance has been one of the major nutritional advice for people with diabetes. However, research has shown that sugars are an integral part of a healthy diet for diabetes, especially sugar gotten from vegetables, fruits, and dairy products. Added sugars, for example, sugar-sweetened and table sugar products, make up around 10% of the day-to-day energy needs. Refined sucrose gives a lower blood glucose reaction than many refined starches. Foods containing sugars vary in physiological effects and nutritional value. For example, sucrose and squeezed orange juice have comparative blood glucose effects but contain different nutrients and minerals. Consuming whole fruits and fruit juices causes blood glucose concentrations to peak slightly earlier but fall more quickly than consuming a comparable carbohydrate portion of white bread.

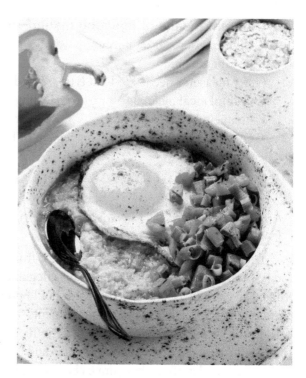

## The Relationship Between Nutrients and Diabetes

People who have diabetes have excess sugar in their blood. Therefore, managing diabetes means managing your blood sugar level through the consumption of food rich in certain nutrients or through insulin injection. The nutrients in what you eat is connected your overall well-being. The right nutrient choices will help you control your blood sugar level. Eating food reach in the right nutrients is one of the primary things you can do to help control diabetes. There isn't one specific "diabetes diet" for people suffering from diabetes. but a dietician can work with you to design a meal plan to guide you on what kinds of food to eat and what snacks to have at mealtimes. A nutritious diet consists of:

- 20% calories from protein
- 40% - 60% from carbohydrates.
- 30% or lesser calories from fat

Your diet should also be low in salt, cholesterol, and added sugar

Contrary to belief eating some sugar doesn't cause problems for most people who have diabetes. However, it's important to watch the amount of sugar you consume and make sure it's part of a balanced diet.

In general, each meal should have the following nutrients:

- 2 - 5 choices (or up to 60 grams) of carbohydrates
- One choice of protein
- A certain amount of fat

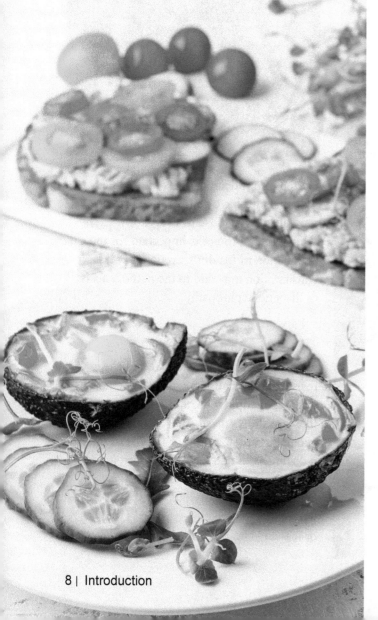

## What to Eat:

- Healthy nuts fats such as almonds, olive oil, walnuts, cashews and peanuts.
- Fresh fruits, vegetables, and whole fruit.
- High-fiber cereals and slices of bread made from whole grains.
- Fish and shellfish.
- Organic chicken or turkey.
- Protein from eggs, low-fat dairy, beans, and unsweetened yogurt.

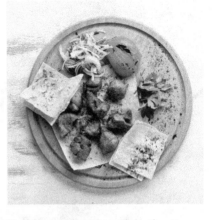

## What to Avoid:

- Processed or fast food, especially those high in sugar.
- Sugary cereals, white bread, refined pasta, or rice.
- Red or processed meat.
- Low-fat products with added sugar, such as fat-free yogurt.

Besides providing diets that will help you manage type 2 diabetes, just like Delicious Dish for Diabetics: Eating Well with Type 2 Diabetes by Robin Ellis, this book offers other benefits as well. The real meat in this book is its use of simple sentences to explain diabetes-related topics such as understand type 2 diabetes, design a menu, how much food should be eaten in a day, food to eat and avoid, and a healthy meal plan for Type 2 diabetes patient. If you are recently diagnosed with Type 2 diabetes, you need a book like this to help get you on the right track for healthy living.

Carbohydrate counting is going to be part of your life now. The recipes in this book are made up of generous amounts of fruits, vegetables, and fiber, which are likely to reduce the risk of cardiovascular diseases and certain types of cancer. The recipes in these book are similar to what you will find in The American Diabetes Association Diabetes Comfort Food Cookbook by Robin Webb, M.S. Embracing a healthy eating plan is the best and fastest way to keep your blood glucose level under control and prevent diabetes complications. Type 2 Diabetics Cookbook for Beginners is here to help you navigate your way around diabetes management by providing a 21-day meal plan made from 200 delicious and healthy recipes to help you develop a good eating habit and ultimately manage your diabetes.

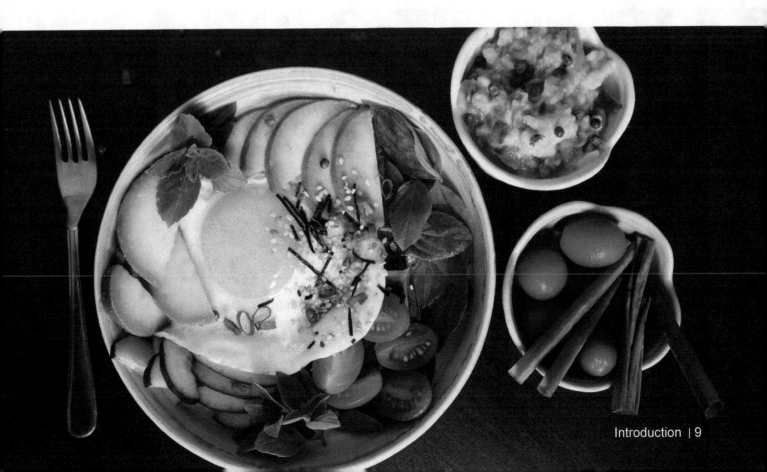

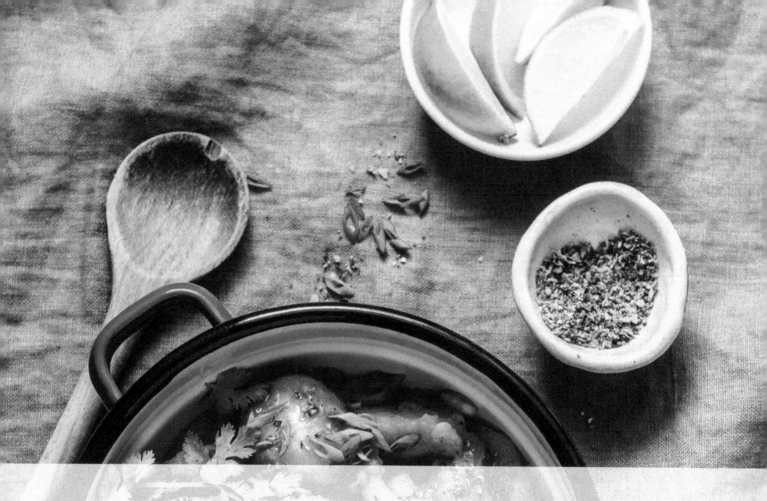

# Chapter 1   Breakfasts

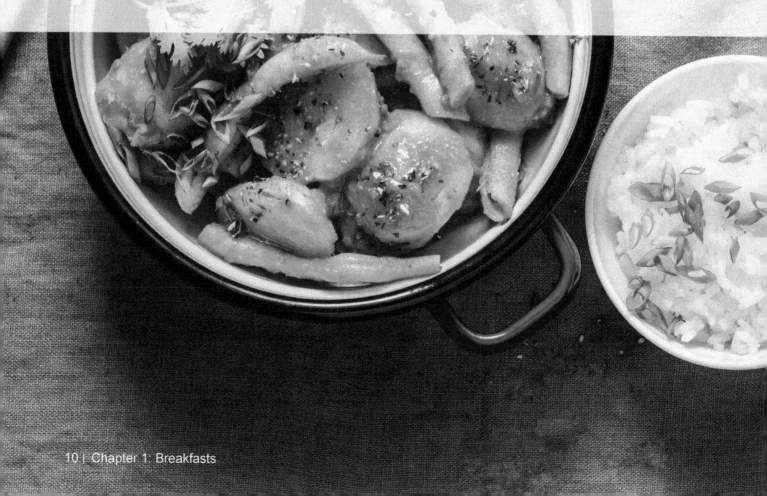

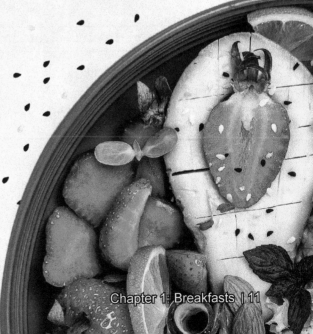

# Breakfast Panini

## Prep time: 10 minutes | Cook time: 10 minutes | Serves 2

2 eggs, beaten
2 tablespoons chopped fresh chives
2 slices tomato
4 ultra-thin slices reduced-sodium deli ham
2 thin slices reduced-fat Cheddar cheese

½ teaspoon salt-free seasoning blend
2 whole wheat thin bagels
2 thin slices onion

1. Spray 8-inch skillet with cooking spray; heat skillet over medium heat. In medium bowl, beat eggs, seasoning and chives with fork or whisk until well mixed. Pour into skillet. As eggs begin to set at bottom and side, gently lift cooked portions with spatula so that thin, uncooked portion can flow to bottom. Avoid constant stirring. Cook 3 to 4 minutes or until eggs are thickened throughout but still moist and creamy; remove from heat. 2. Meanwhile, heat closed contact grill or panini maker 5 minutes. 3. For each panini, divide cooked eggs evenly between bottom halves of bagels. Top each with 1 slice each tomato and onion, 2 ham slices, 1 cheese slice and top half of bagel. Transfer filled panini to heated grill. Close cover, pressing down lightly. Cook 2 to 3 minutes or until browned and cheese is melted. Serve immediately.

**Per Serving**

Calories: 260 | fat: 7g | protein: 15g | carbs: 32g | sugars: 5g | fiber: 2g | sodium: 410mg

# Orange-Berry Pancake Syrup

## Prep time: 5 minutes | Cook time: 0 minutes | Serves 8

2 cups raspberries, fresh or frozen
¼ cup pure maple syrup

½ cup fresh orange juice
Pinch of sea salt

1. In a blender, combine the raspberries, juice, syrup, and salt. Puree until smooth, stopping to scrape down the blender as needed. If the mixture is too thick (particularly if using frozen berries), you may need to scrape down more often or add a tablespoon or two of water to assist with the blending. Once it's smooth, transfer the syrup to a jar or other airtight container and store it in the refrigerator. It keeps for about a week in the fridge.

**Per Serving**

Calorie: 65 | fat: 0.4g | protein: 1g | carbs: 16g | sugars: 10g | fiber: 4g | sodium: 38mg

# Sweet Potato Toasts

## Prep time: 10 minutes | Cook time: 2 minutes | Serves 1

2 slices sprouted grain bread
½–1 teaspoon lemon juice
Freshly ground black pepper (optional)

½ cup mashed cooked sweet potato, peel removed
A couple pinches of sea salt
2 tablespoons cubed avocado or
1 tablespoon sliced black olives

1. Toast the bread. In a small bowl, mash the sweet potato with the lemon juice (adjusting to taste), salt, and pepper (if using). Distribute the mashed sweet potato between the slices of toast, and top with either the cubed avocado or the black olives. Serve!

**Per Serving**

Calorie: 312 | fat: 5g | protein: 8g | carbs: 59g | sugars: 11g | fiber: 8g | sodium: 1018mg

# Potato, Egg and Sausage Frittata

## Prep time: 30 minutes | Cook time: 20 minutes | Serves 4

4 frozen soy-protein breakfast sausage links (from 8-ounce box), thawed
4 eggs or 8 egg whites
¼ cup fat-free (skim) milk
⅛ teaspoon dried basil leaves
1½ cups chopped plum (Roma) tomatoes
Pepper, if desired
Chopped green onion, if desired

1 teaspoon olive oil
2 cups frozen country-style shredded hash brown potatoes (from 30-ounce bag)
¼ teaspoon salt
⅛ teaspoon dried oregano leaves
½ cup shredded mozzarella and Asiago cheese blend with garlic (2 ounces)

1. Cut each sausage link into 8 pieces. Coat 10-inch nonstick skillet with oil; heat over medium heat. Add sausage and potatoes; cook 6 to 8 minutes, stirring occasionally, until potatoes are golden brown. 2. In small bowl, beat eggs and milk with fork or whisk until well blended. Pour egg mixture over potato mixture. Cook uncovered over medium-low heat about 5 minutes; as mixture begins to set on bottom and side, gently lift cooked portions with spatula so that thin, uncooked portion can flow to bottom. Cook until eggs are thickened throughout but still moist; avoid constant stirring. 3. Sprinkle salt, basil, oregano, tomatoes and cheese over eggs. Reduce heat to low; cover and cook about 5 minutes or until center is set and cheese is melted. Sprinkle with pepper and green onion.

**Per Serving**
Calorie: 280 | fat: 12g | protein: 17g | carbs: 26g | sugars: 5g | fiber: 3g | sodium: 590mg

# Grain-Free Apple Cinnamon Cake

## Prep time: 10 minutes | Cook time: 50 minutes | Serves 8

2 cups almond flour
1½ teaspoons ground cinnamon
½ teaspoon fine sea salt
2 large eggs
1 small apple, chopped into small pieces

½ cup Lakanto Monkfruit Sweetener Golden
1 teaspoon baking powder
½ cup plain 2 percent Greek yogurt
½ teaspoon pure vanilla extract

1. Pour 1 cup water into the Instant Pot. Line the base of a 7 by 3-inch round cake pan with parchment paper. Butter the sides of the pan and the parchment or coat with nonstick cooking spray. 2. In a medium bowl, whisk together the almond flour, sweetener, cinnamon, baking powder, and salt. In a smaller bowl, whisk together the yogurt, eggs, and vanilla until no streaks of yolk remain. Add the wet mixture to the dry mixture and stir just until the dry ingredients are evenly moistened, then fold in the apple. The batter will be very thick. 3. Transfer the batter to the prepared pan and, using a rubber spatula, spread it in an even layer. Cover the pan tightly with aluminum foil. Place the pan on a long-handled silicone steam rack, then, holding the handles of the steam rack, lower it into the Instant Pot. (If you don't have the long-handled rack, use the wire metal steam rack and a homemade sling) 4. Secure the lid and set the Pressure Release to Sealing. Select the Cake, Pressure Cook, or Manual setting and set the cooking time for 40 minutes at high pressure. (The pot will take about 10 minutes to come up to pressure before the cooking program begins.) 5. When the cooking program ends, let the pressure release naturally for 10 minutes, then move the Pressure Release to Venting to release any remaining steam. Open the pot and, wearing heat-resistant mitts, grasp the handles of the steam rack and lift it out of the pot. Uncover the pan, taking care not to get burned by the steam or to drip condensation onto the cake. Let the cake cool in the pan on a cooling rack for about 5 minutes. 6. Run a butter knife around the edge of the pan to loosen the cake from the pan sides. Invert the cake onto the rack, lift off the pan, and peel off the parchment. Let cool for 15 minutes, then invert the cake onto a serving plate. Cut into eight wedges and serve.

**Per Serving**
Calories: 219 | fat: 16g | protein: 9g | carbs: 20g | sugars: 8g | fiber: 16g | sodium: 154mg

# Instant Pot Hard-Boiled Eggs

## Prep time: 10 minutes | Cook time: 5 minutes | Serves 7

1 cup water                                             6–8 eggs

1. Pour the water into the inner pot. Place the eggs in a steamer basket or rack that came with pot. 2. Close the lid and secure to the locking position. Be sure the vent is turned to sealing. Set for 5 minutes on Manual at high pressure. (It takes about 5 minutes for pressure to build and then 5 minutes to cook.) 3. Let pressure naturally release for 5 minutes, then do quick pressure release. 4. Place hot eggs into cool water to halt cooking process. You can peel cooled eggs immediately or refrigerate unpeeled.

**Per Serving**
Calories: 72 | fat: 5g | protein: 6g | carbs: 0g | sugars: 0g | fiber: 0g | sodium: 71mg

# Tropical Fruit 'n Ginger Oatmeal

## Prep time: 15 minutes | Cook time: 25 to 30 minutes | Serves 4

2¼ cups water                                           ¾ cup steel-cut oats
2 teaspoons finely chopped gingerroot                   ⅛ teaspoon salt
½ medium banana, mashed                                 1 container (6 ounces) vanilla low-fat yogurt
1 medium mango, pitted, peeled and chopped (1 cup)      ½ cup sliced fresh strawberries
2 tablespoons shredded coconut, toasted                 2 tablespoons chopped walnuts

In 1½-quart saucepan, heat water to boiling. Stir in oats, gingerroot and salt. Reduce heat; simmer gently uncovered 25 to 30 minutes, without stirring, until oats are tender yet slightly chewy; stir in banana. Divide oatmeal evenly among 4 bowls. 2. Top each serving with yogurt, mango, strawberries, coconut and walnuts. Serve immediately.

**Per Serving**
Calories: 200 | fat: 6g | protein: 5g | carbs: 31g | sugars: 16g | fiber: 4g | sodium: 110mg

# Corn, Egg and Potato Bake

## Prep time: 20 minutes | Cook time: 1 hour | Serves 8

4 cups frozen diced hash brown potatoes (from 2-pound bag), thawed
½ cup frozen whole-kernel corn (from 1-pound bag), thawed
¼ cup chopped roasted red bell peppers (from 7-ounce jar)
1½ cups shredded reduced-fat Colby–Monterey Jack cheese (6 ounces)
10 eggs or 2½ cups fat-free egg product
½ cup fat-free small-curd cottage cheese
½ teaspoon dried oregano leaves
¼ teaspoon garlic powder
4 medium green onions, chopped (¼ cup)

Heat oven to 350°F. Spray 11x7-inch (2-quart) glass baking dish with cooking spray. In baking dish, layer potatoes, corn, bell peppers and 1 cup of the shredded cheese. 2. In medium bowl, beat eggs, cottage cheese, oregano and garlic powder with whisk until well blended. Slowly pour over potato mixture. Sprinkle with onions and remaining ½ cup shredded cheese. 3. Cover and bake 30 minutes. Uncover and bake about 30 minutes longer or until knife inserted in center comes out clean. Let stand 5 to 10 minutes before cutting.

**Per Serving**
Calories: 240 | fat: 11g | protein: 16g | carbs: 18g | sugars: 2g | fiber: 2g | sodium: 440mg

# Crustless Potato, Spinach, and Mushroom Quiche

### Prep time: 10 minutes | Cook time: 40 minutes | Serves 4

8 ounces yellow potatoes, thinly sliced

2 teaspoons dried thyme, divided

10 ounces button mushrooms, coarsely chopped

2 cups baby spinach

2 cups 1% milk

½ cup julienned sun-dried tomatoes (see Tip)

1 tablespoon olive oil

1 teaspoon dried rosemary

1 teaspoon balsamic vinegar

6 large eggs

2 ounces goat cheese, crumbled

1. Preheat the oven to 375°F (191°C). 2. In a large bowl, toss the potatoes with the oil, 1 teaspoon of the thyme, and rosemary. Arrange the potatoes on the bottom of a large oven-safe skillet or baking dish. Bake the potatoes for 10 to 15 minutes, or until they soften and start to crisp. Do not turn off the oven. 3. Meanwhile, combine the remaining 1 teaspoon of thyme and the mushrooms in a large skillet over medium-high heat. Cook the mushrooms for about 5 minutes, or until the mushrooms are brown and most of their liquid has evaporated. Stir in the vinegar. Add the spinach and cook it for 3 to 4 minutes, stirring constantly, until it is wilted. Remove the mushrooms and spinach from the heat and set them aside. 4. In a large bowl, whisk together the eggs and milk. Add the mushroom and spinach mixture, goat cheese, and sun-dried tomatoes. Pour the mixture into the potato-lined skillet and bake the quiche for 25 minutes, or until the eggs are set and no longer runny in the center.

**Per Serving**

Calorie: 322 | fat: 16g | protein: 22g | carbs: 25g | sugars: 12g | fiber: 3g | sodium: 218mg

# Coddled Huevos Rancheros

### Prep time: 5 minutes | Cook time: 10 minutes | Serves 2

2 teaspoons unsalted butter

1 cup drained cooked black beans, or two-thirds

15-ounce can black beans, rinsed and drained

2 cups shredded romaine lettuce

2 tablespoons grated Cotija cheese

4 large eggs

Two 7-inch corn or whole-wheat tortillas, warmed

½ cup chunky tomato salsa (such as Pace brand)

1 tablespoon chopped fresh cilantro

1. Pour 1 cup water into the Instant Pot and place a long-handled silicone steam rack into the pot. (If you don't have the long-handled rack, use the wire metal steam rack and a homemade sling) 2. Coat each of four 4-ounce ramekins with ½ teaspoon butter. Crack an egg into each ramekin. Place the ramekins on the steam rack in the pot. 3. Secure the lid and set the Pressure Release to Sealing. Select the Steam setting and set the cooking time for 3 minutes at low pressure. (The pot will take about 5 minutes to come up to pressure before the cooking program begins.) 4. While the eggs are cooking, in a small saucepan over low heat, warm the beans for about 5 minutes, stirring occasionally. Cover the saucepan and remove from the heat. (Alternatively, warm the beans in a covered bowl in a microwave for 1 minute. Leave the beans covered until ready to serve.) 5. When the cooking program ends, let the pressure release naturally for 5 minutes, then move the Pressure Release to Venting to release any remaining steam. Open the pot and, wearing heat-resistant mitts, grasp the handles of the steam rack and carefully lift it out of the pot. 6. Place a warmed tortilla on each plate and spoon ½ cup of the beans onto each tortilla. Run a knife around the inside edge of each ramekin to loosen the egg and unmold two eggs onto the beans on each tortilla. Spoon the salsa over the eggs and top with the lettuce, cilantro, and cheese. Serve right away.

**Per Serving**

Calorie: 112 | fat: 8g | protein: 8g | carbs: 3g | sugars: 0g | fiber: 0g | sodium: 297mg

# Peaches and Cream Yogurt Bowl

## Prep time: 5 minutes | Cook time: 0 minutes | Serves 1

6 ounces (170 g) plain Greek yogurt
½ teaspoon ground cinnamon
1 tablespoon almond butter
1 teaspoon honey (optional)

½ teaspoon pure vanilla extract
1 medium peach, sliced to desired thickness,
or 1 cup (250 g) frozen sliced peaches

1. In a small bowl, stir together the yogurt, vanilla, and cinnamon. Add the peach slices and drizzle the yogurt bowl with the almond butter and honey (if using).
**Per Serving**
Calorie: 361 | fat: 19g | protein: 24g | carbs: 27g | sugars: 21g | fiber: 6g | sodium: 91mg

# Green Nice Cream Breakfast Bowl

## Prep time: 5 minutes | Cook time: 0 minutes | Serves 3

3 cups sliced, frozen, overripe banana
2 cups baby spinach
Pinch of sea salt
1–2 tablespoons coconut syrup (optional)
½ cup fresh berries

1 cup frozen pineapple chunks
Flesh of 1 ripe avocado (about ½ cup)
3–5 tablespoons low-fat nondairy milk
½ cup fresh sliced banana

1. In a blender or food processor, combine the banana, pineapple, spinach, avocado, salt, and 3 tablespoons of the milk. Puree until very smooth. If the mixture is stubborn and not blending, add the additional 2 tablespoons of milk as needed to get the mixture moving. Taste, and add the syrup if desired to sweeten. Spoon the mixture into 3 serving bowls, and top with the banana and berries.
**Per Serving**
Calorie: 337 | fat: 8g | protein: 5g | carbs: 70g | sugars: 37g | fiber: 12g | sodium: 126mg

# Easy Sweet Potato and Egg Sandwiches

## Prep time: 5 minutes | Cook time: 10 minutes | Serves 2

1 large sweet potato, sliced into
4 (¼-inch [6-mm]-thick) rounds
2 large eggs

2 ounces (57 g) shredded mozzarella cheese
Cooking oil spray, as needed

1. Preheat the oven to broil. Line a large baking sheet with parchment paper. 2. Arrange the sweet potato rounds evenly on the prepared baking sheet. Broil the sweet potatoes for 4 to 6 minutes, until they are beginning to brown. Make sure to keep an eye on them so they don't burn. 3. Remove the sweet potatoes from the oven and add 1 ounce (28 g) of mozzarella cheese per sweet potato round to two of the rounds. Remove the plain sweet potato rounds from the baking sheet, and return the baking sheet with the cheese-topped sweet potatoes to the oven. Broil the rounds for 1 to 2 minutes, until the cheese begins to brown. 4. Remove the baking sheet from the oven and set it aside with the other sweet potato rounds. 5. Heat a medium skillet over medium heat. Spray it with the cooking oil spray and add the eggs. Scramble the eggs to your preferred doneness. 6. Top the cheesy sweet potato rounds with some of the scrambled eggs and the remaining sweet potato rounds. Slice the sandwiches and serve them.
**Per Serving**
Calorie: 222 | fat: 9g | protein: 15g | carbs: 20g | sugars: 4g | fiber: 3g | sodium: 297mg

# Overnight Berry Oats

### Prep time: 5 minutes | Cook time: 0 minutes | Serves 2

1 cup rolled oats
1 cup raspberries or mixed berries (such as blueberries, strawberries, and blackberries), fresh or frozen
1 cup and 1–2 tablespoons low-fat nondairy milk (plus more for serving, if desired)
½ tablespoon chia seeds
2 tablespoons coconut nectar or pure maple syrup
Pinch of sea salt

1. In a bowl or large jar, combine the oats, berries, milk, chia seeds, nectar or syrup, and salt. Cover and refrigerate overnight (or for at least several hours). Serve with more milk to thin, if desired, and also try some additional add-ins.

**Per Serving**

Calorie: 326 | fat: 5g | protein: 9g | carbs: 64g | sugars: 21g | fiber: 14g | sodium: 205mg

# Sunrise Smoothie Bowl

### Prep time: 5 minutes | Cook time: 0 minutes | Serves 1

½ cup frozen raspberries
½ large banana
½ cup plain nonfat Greek yogurt
1 tablespoon unsweetened coconut flakes

½ cup frozen strawberries
½ cup cauliflower florets
Water, as needed
2 tablespoons coarsely chopped walnuts

1. In a high-power blender, combine the raspberries, strawberries, banana, cauliflower, and yogurt. Blend the ingredients until they are smooth, adding water as needed to reach the desired consistency. 2. Pour the smoothie into a bowl and top it with the coconut flakes and walnuts.

**Per Serving**

Calorie: 336 | fat: 14g | protein: 17g | carbs: 44g | sugars: 21g | fiber: 12g | sodium: 69mg

# Baked Eggs

### Prep time: 15 minutes | Cook time: 20 minutes | Serves 8

1 cup water
1 cup reduced-fat buttermilk baking mix
2 teaspoons chopped onion
½ cup grated reduced-fat cheddar cheese
1¼ cups egg substitute

2 tablespoons no-trans-fat tub margarine, melted
1½ cups fat-free cottage cheese
1 teaspoon dried parsley
1 egg, slightly beaten
1 cup fat-free milk

1. Place the steaming rack into the bottom of the inner pot and pour in 1 cup of water. 2. Grease a round springform pan that will fit into the inner pot of the Instant Pot. 3. Pour melted margarine into springform pan. 4. Mix together buttermilk baking mix, cottage cheese, onion, parsley, cheese, egg, egg substitute, and milk in large mixing bowl. 5. Pour mixture over melted margarine. Stir slightly to distribute margarine. 6. Place the springform pan onto the steaming rack, close the lid, and secure to the locking position. Be sure the vent is turned to sealing. Set for 20 minutes on Manual at high pressure. 7. Let the pressure release naturally. 8. Carefully remove the springform pan with the handles of the steaming rack and allow to stand 10 minutes before cutting and serving.

**Per Serving**

Calories: 155 | fat: 5g | protein: 12g | carbs: 15g | sugars: 4g | fiber: 0g | sodium: 460mg

# Double-Berry Muffins

**Prep time: 15 minutes | Cook time: 20 to 25 minutes | Makes 12 muffins**

¼ cup packed brown sugar
1 cup fat-free (skim) milk
2 tablespoons canola oil
1 egg or ¼ cup fat-free egg product
⅓ cup granulated sugar
½ teaspoon salt
½ cup fresh or frozen (thawed and drained) blueberries

½ teaspoon ground cinnamon
¼ cup unsweetened applesauce
½ teaspoon vanilla
2 cups all-purpose flour
3 teaspoons baking powder
½ cup fresh or frozen (thawed and drained) raspberries

1. Heat oven to 400°F. Place paper baking cup in each of 12 regular-size muffin cups, or grease bottoms only with shortening. In small bowl, mix brown sugar and cinnamon; set aside. 2. In large bowl, beat milk, applesauce, oil, vanilla and egg with fork or whisk. Stir in flour, granulated sugar, baking powder and salt all at once just until flour is moistened (batter will be lumpy). Fold in raspberries and blueberries. Divide batter evenly among muffin cups. Sprinkle brown sugar mixture evenly over tops of muffins. 3. Bake 20 to 25 minutes or until golden brown. Immediately remove from pan to cooling rack. Serve warm if desired.

**Per Serving**
Calories: 160 | fat: 3g | protein: 3g | carbs: 30g | sugars: 12g | fiber: 1g | sodium: 240mg

# Cinnamon Wisp Pancakes

**Prep time: 5 minutes | Cook time: 10 minutes | Serves 4**

2 cups oat flour
1 tablespoon baking powder
Pinch of sea salt
1¾ cups + ¼ cup vanilla low-fat nondairy milk

2 tablespoons chia seeds
2 teaspoons cinnamon
1½ teaspoons vanilla extract

1. In a large bowl, combine the oat flour, chia seeds, baking powder, cinnamon, and salt. Stir to combine. Add the vanilla and 1¾ cups of the milk, and whisk through the dry mixture until combined. Let the batter sit for a few minutes to thicken. 2. Lightly coat a large nonstick skillet with cooking spray. Heat the pan over medium-high heat for a few minutes until hot, then reduce the heat to medium or medium-low and let it rest for a minute. Using a ladle, scoop ¼ to ⅓ cup of the batter into the pan for each pancake. Depending on the size of pan, cook 2 or 3 pancakes at a time. Cook for several minutes, until small bubbles form on the outer edges and in the centers and the pancakes start to look dry on the top. (Wait until those bubbles form, or the pancakes will be tricky to flip.) Once ready, flip the pancakes to lightly cook the other side for about a minute. Repeat until the batter is all used, adding the extra milk, 1 tablespoon at a time, if needed to thin the batter as you go.

**Per Serving**
Calorie: 312 | fat: 6g | protein: 11g | carbs: 54g | sugars: 5g | fiber: 9g | sodium: 483mg

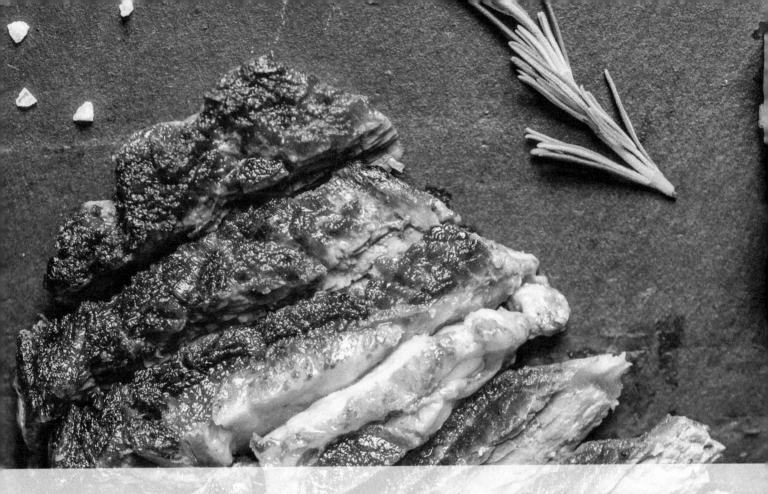

# Chapter 2 Beef, Pork, and Lamb

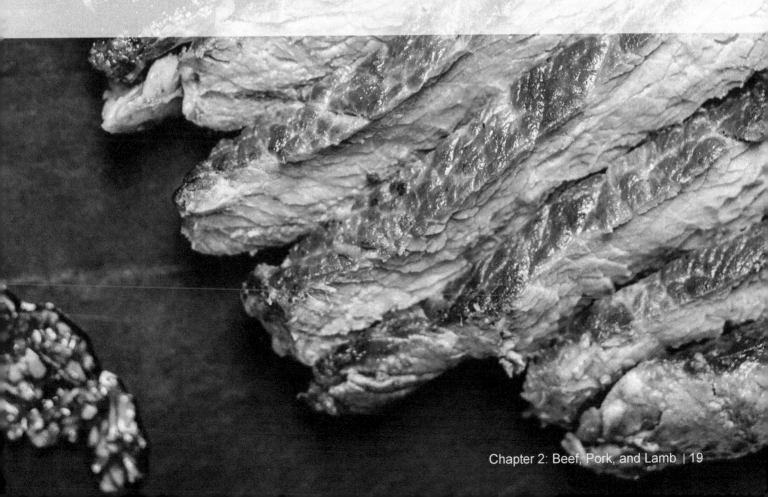

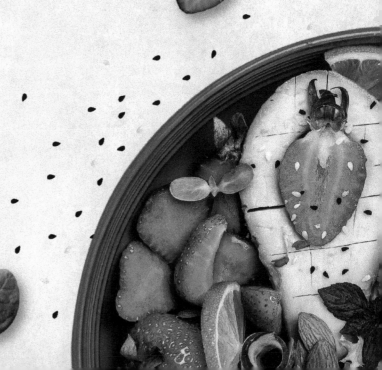

# Pork Chops with Raspberry-Chipotle Sauce and Herbed Rice

## Prep time: 25 minutes | Cook time: 10 minutes | Serves 4

### Pork Chops

4 bone-in pork rib chops, about ¾ inch thick
1 tablespoon canola oil
⅓ cup all-fruit raspberry spread
1 tablespoon raspberry-flavored vinegar
1 large or 2 small chipotle chiles in adobo sauce,

½ teaspoon garlic-pepper blend
Raspberry-Chipotle Sauce
1 tablespoon water
finely chopped (from 7-ounce can)

### Herbed Rice

1 package (8.8 ounces) quick-cooking (ready in 90 seconds) whole-grain brown rice
1 tablespoon chopped fresh cilantro

¼ teaspoon salt-free garlic-herb blend
½ teaspoon lemon peel

1. Sprinkle pork with garlic pepper. In 12-inch nonstick skillet, heat oil over medium-high heat. Add pork to oil. Cook 8 to 10 minutes, turning once, until pork is no longer pink and meat thermometer inserted in center reads 145°F. Remove from skillet to serving platter (reserve pork drippings); keep warm. 2. Meanwhile, in small bowl, stir raspberry spread, water, vinegar and chile; set aside. Make rice as directed on package. Stir in remaining rice ingredients; keep warm. 3 In skillet with pork drippings, pour raspberry mixture. Cook and stir over low heat about 1 minute or until sauce is bubbly and slightly thickened. Serve pork chops with sauce and rice.

**Per Serving**
Calories: 370 | fat: 12g | protein: 31g | carbs: 34g | sugars: 12g | fiber: 0g | sodium: 140mg

# Ground Beef Tacos

## Prep time: 0 minutes | Cook time: 25 minutes | Serves 6

### Filling

1 tablespoon cold-pressed avocado oil or other neutral oil
1½ pounds 95 percent lean ground beef
½ cup low-sodium roasted beef bone broth

2 garlic cloves, minced
1 yellow onion, diced
2 tablespoons chili powder

### Fine sea salt

1 tablespoon tomato paste
1 cup chopped white onion
2 tablespoons chopped fresh cilantro
Hot sauce (such as Cholula or Tapatío) for serving

Twelve 7-inch corn tortillas, warmed
1 cup chopped tomatoes
1 large avocado, pitted, peeled, and sliced

1. To make the filling: Select the Sauté setting on the Instant Pot and heat the oil and garlic for 2 minutes, until the garlic is bubbling but not browned. Add the yellow onion and sauté for about 3 minutes, until it begins to soften. Add the ground beef and sauté, using a wooden spoon or spatula to break up the meat as it cooks for about 3 minutes more; it's fine if some streaks of pink remain, the beef does not need to be cooked through. Stir in the chili powder, bone broth, and ½ teaspoon salt. Dollop the tomato paste on top. Do not stir it in. 2. Secure the lid and set the Pressure Release to Sealing. Press the Cancel button to reset the cooking program, then select the Pressure Cook or Manual setting and set the cooking time for 10 minutes at high pressure. (The pot will take about 5 minutes to come up to pressure before the cooking program begins.) 3. When the cooking program ends, you can either perform a quick pressure release by moving the Pressure Release to Venting, or you can let the pressure release naturally and leave the pot on the Keep Warm setting for up to 10 hours. Open the pot and give the meat a stir. Taste for seasoning and add more salt, if needed. 4. Using a slotted spoon, spoon the meat onto the tortillas. Top with the white onion, tomatoes, cilantro, and avocado and serve right away. Pass the hot sauce at the table.

**Per Serving**
Calories: 353 | fat: 13g | protein: 28g | carbs: 28g | sugars: 3g | fiber: 6g | sodium: 613mg

# Couscous and Sweet Potatoes with Pork

## Prep time: 20 minutes | Cook time: 10 minutes | Serves 5

1¼ cups uncooked couscous
1 medium sweet potato, peeled, cut into julienne strips
½ cup water
¼ cup chopped fresh cilantro

1 pound pork tenderloin, thinly sliced
1 cup chunky-style salsa
2 tablespoons honey

1. Cook couscous as directed on package. 2. While couscous is cooking, spray 12-inch skillet with cooking spray. Cook pork in skillet over medium heat 2 to 3 minutes, stirring occasionally, until brown. 3. Stir sweet potato, salsa, water and honey into pork. Heat to boiling; reduce heat to medium. Cover and cook 5 to 6 minutes, stirring occasionally, until potato is tender. Sprinkle with cilantro. Serve pork mixture over couscous.

**Per Serving**

Calorie: 320 | fat: 4g | protein: 23g | carbs: 48g | sugars: 11g | fiber: 3g | sodium: 420mg

# Shepherd's Pie with Cauliflower-Carrot Mash

## Prep time: 10 minutes | Cook time: 35 minutes | Serves 6

1 tablespoon coconut oil
1 large yellow onion, diced
1 pound 95 percent lean ground beef
1 teaspoons dried thyme
1 teaspoon freshly ground black pepper
2 tablespoons Worcestershire sauce
3 tablespoons tomato paste
1 pound cauliflower florets
¼ cup coconut milk or other nondairy milk
½ cup sliced green onions, white and green parts

2 garlic cloves, minced
1 pound ground lamb
½ cup low-sodium vegetable broth
1 teaspoon dried sage
1¾ teaspoons fine sea salt
One 12-ounce bag frozen baby lima beans, green peas, or shelled edamame
1 pound carrots, halved lengthwise and then crosswise (or quartered if very large)

1. Select the Sauté setting on the Instant Pot and heat the oil and garlic for 2 minutes, until the garlic is bubbling but not browned. Add the onion and sauté for 3 minutes, until it begins to soften. Add the lamb and beef and sauté, using a wooden spoon or spatula to break up the meat as it cooks, for 6 minutes, until cooked through and no streaks of pink remain. 2. Stir in the broth, using the spoon or spatula to nudge any browned bits from the bottom of the pot. Add the thyme, sage, pepper, ¾ teaspoon of the salt, the Worcestershire sauce, and lima beans and stir to mix. Dollop the tomato paste on top. Do not stir it in. 3. Place a tall steam rack in the pot, then place the cauliflower and carrots on top of the rack. 4. Secure the lid and set the Pressure Release to Sealing. Press the Cancel button to reset the cooking program, then select the Pressure Cook or Manual setting and set the cooking time for 4 minutes at low pressure. (The pot will take about 15 minutes to come up to pressure before the cooking program begins.) 5. Position an oven rack 4 to 6 inches below the heat source and preheat the broiler. 6. When the cooking program ends, perform a quick pressure release by moving the Pressure Release to Venting. Open the pot and, using tongs, transfer the cauliflower and carrots to a bowl. Add the coconut milk and remaining 1 teaspoon salt to the bowl. Using an immersion blender, blend the vegetables until smooth. 7. Wearing heat-resistant mitts, remove the steam rack from the pot. Stir ½ cup of the mashed vegetables into the filling mixture in the pot, incorporating the tomato paste at the same time. Remove the inner pot from the housing. Transfer the mixture to a broiler-safe 9 by 13-inch baking dish, spreading it in an even layer. Dollop the mashed vegetables on top and spread them out evenly with a fork. Broil, checking often, for 5 to 8 minutes, until the mashed vegetables are lightly browned. 8. Spoon the shepherd's pie onto plates, sprinkle with the green onions, and serve hot.

**Per Serving**

Calories: 437 | fat: 18g | protein: 39g | carbs: 33g | sugars: 8g | fiber: 9g | sodium: 802mg

# Parmesan-Crusted Pork Chops

## Prep time: 5 minutes | Cook time: 12 minutes | Serves 4

1 large egg
4 (4-ounce / 113-g) boneless pork chops
¼ teaspoon ground black pepper

½ cup grated Parmesan cheese
½ teaspoon salt

1. Whisk egg in a medium bowl and place Parmesan in a separate medium bowl. 2. Sprinkle pork chops on both sides with salt and pepper. Dip each pork chop into egg, then press both sides into Parmesan. 3. Place pork chops into ungreased air fryer basket. Adjust the temperature to 400°F (204°C) and air fry for 12 minutes, turning chops halfway through cooking. Pork chops will be golden and have an internal temperature of at least 145°F (63°C) when done. Serve warm.

**Per Serving**
Calories: 332 | fat: 16g | protein: 44g | carbs: 1g | sugars: 0g | fiber: 0g | sodium: 440mg

# Salisbury Steaks with Seared Cauliflower

## Prep time: 5 minutes | Cook time: 30 minutes | Serves 4

**Salisbury Steaks**
1 pound 95 percent lean ground beef
1 large egg
¼ teaspoon freshly ground black pepper
1 small yellow onion, sliced
8 ounces cremini or button mushrooms, sliced
2 tablespoons tomato paste
1 cup low-sodium roasted beef bone broth

⅓ cup almond flour
½ teaspoon fine sea salt
2 tablespoons cold-pressed avocado oil
1 garlic clove, chopped
½ teaspoon fine sea salt
1½ teaspoons yellow mustard

**Seared Cauliflower**
1 tablespoon olive oil
2 tablespoons chopped fresh flat-leaf parsley
2 teaspoons cornstarch

1 head cauliflower, cut into bite-size florets
¼ teaspoon fine sea salt
2 teaspoons water

**To make the steaks:**
In a bowl, combine the beef, almond flour, egg, salt, and pepper and mix with your hands until all of the ingredients are evenly distributed. Divide the mixture into four equal portions, then shape each portion into an oval patty about ½ inch thick. 2. Select the Sauté setting on the Instant Pot and heat the oil for 2 minutes. Swirl the oil to coat the bottom of the pot, then add the patties and sear for 3 minutes, until browned on one side. Using a thin, flexible spatula, flip the patties and sear the second side for 2 to 3 minutes, until browned. Transfer the patties to a plate. 3. Add the onion, garlic, mushrooms, and salt to the pot and sauté for 4 minutes, until the onion is translucent and the mushrooms have begun to give up their liquid. Add the tomato paste, mustard, and broth and stir with a wooden spoon, using it to nudge any browned bits from the bottom of the pot. Return the patties to the pot in a single layer and spoon a bit of the sauce over each one. 4. Secure the lid and set the Pressure Release to Sealing. Press the Cancel button to reset the cooking program, then select the Pressure Cook or Manual setting and set the cooking time for 10 minutes at high pressure. (The pot will take about 5 minutes to come up to pressure before the cooking program begins.) 5. When the cooking program ends, let the pressure release naturally for at least 10 minutes, then move the Pressure Release to Venting to release any remaining steam.
To make the cauliflower: 1. While the pressure is releasing, in a large skillet over medium heat, warm the oil. Add the cauliflower and stir or toss to coat with the oil, then cook, stirring every minute or two, until lightly browned, about 8 minutes. Turn off the heat, sprinkle in the parsley and salt, and stir to combine. Leave in the skillet, uncovered, to keep warm. 2. Open the pot and, using a slotted spatula, transfer the patties to a serving plate. In a small bowl, stir together the cornstarch and water. Press the Cancel button to reset the cooking program, then select the Sauté setting. When the sauce comes to a simmer, stir in the cornstarch mixture and let the sauce boil for about 1 minute, until thickened. Press the Cancel button to turn off the Instant Pot. 3. Spoon the sauce over the patties. Serve right away, with the cauliflower.

**Per Serving**
Calorie: 362 | fat: 21g | protein: 33g | carbs: 21g | sugars: 4g | fiber: 6g | sodium: 846mg

# Slow Cooker Chipotle Beef Stew

## Prep time: 25 minutes | Cook time: 8 to 10 hours | Serves 6

### Stew

1 package (12 ounces) frozen whole kernel corn

1 chipotle chile in adobo sauce (from 7-ounce can), finely chopped

2 poblano chiles, seeded, diced

2 cans (14.5 ounces each) diced tomatoes, undrained

½ teaspoon salt

1 pound boneless beef top sirloin, trimmed of fat, cut into 1-inch cubes

2 large onions, chopped (2 cups)

3 cloves garlic, chopped

1½ teaspoons ground cumin

¼ teaspoon cracked black pepper

### Toppings

1 avocado, pitted, peeled cut into 12 wedges

6 small cilantro sprigs, coarsely chopped

12 baked tortilla chips, crushed

6 tablespoons reduced-fat sour cream

1. Spray 4- to 5-quart slow cooker with cooking spray. In small microwavable bowl, microwave corn uncovered on High 2 minutes or until thawed. In slow cooker, place corn and all remaining stew ingredients; mix well. Cover and cook on Low heat setting 8 to 10 hours (or High heat setting 4 to 5 hours). 2. Divide stew evenly among 6 bowls. To serve, top with avocado, tortilla chips, cilantro and sour cream.

**Per Serving**

Calories: 310 | fat: 10g | protein: 25g | carbs: 30g | sugars: 10g | fiber: 5g | sodium: 580mg

# Pork Mole Quesadillas

## Prep time: 35 minutes | Cook time: 15 minutes | Makes 4 quesadillas

2 teaspoons canola oil

1 medium green bell pepper, thinly sliced

1 medium red bell pepper, thinly sliced

3 cloves garlic, finely chopped

1 teaspoon all-purpose flour

¼ teaspoon salt

¼ cup reduced-sodium chicken broth

4 fat-free flour tortillas (10 inch)

½ pound boneless pork loin chops, trimmed of fat, cut into thin strips

1 medium onion, thinly sliced

1 tablespoon chili powder

1 teaspoon ground cumin

¼ teaspoon ground cinnamon

2 tablespoons semisweet chocolate chips

### Cooking spray

½ cup chopped tomato

½ cup shredded reduced-fat Monterey Jack cheese (2 ounces)

4 teaspoons chopped fresh cilantro

1. In 12-inch nonstick skillet, heat 1 teaspoon of the oil over medium-high heat. Add pork to oil. Cook 4 to 5 minutes, stirring frequently, until pork is no longer pink; remove from skillet. 2. In same skillet, heat remaining 1 teaspoon oil over medium heat. Add bell peppers, onion and garlic to oil. Cook 3 to 5 minutes, stirring occasionally, until bell peppers are crisp-tender. Stir in chili powder, flour, cumin, salt and cinnamon; cook 30 seconds. Stir in chicken broth; heat to boiling. Cook about 30 seconds, stirring constantly, until thickened and bubbly. Remove from heat; stir in chocolate chips until melted. Stir in pork. 3. Spray 1 side of each tortilla with cooking spray. On work surface, place tortillas, sprayed side down. Arrange pork mixture, tomato, cilantro and cheese evenly over half of each tortilla. Fold tortilla over filling, pressing gently. 4. Heat 12-inch skillet over medium heat until hot. Cook 2 quesadillas 3 to 4 minutes, turning once, until tortillas begin to brown; remove quesadillas from pan. Keep warm. Repeat with remaining 2 quesadillas. 5. To serve, cut into wedges, beginning from center of folded side.

**Per Serving**

Calories: 450 | fat: 17g | protein: 23g | carbs: 50g | sugars: 8g | fiber: 4g | sodium: 810mg

# Carnitas Burrito Bowls

**Prep time: 10 minutes | Cook time: 1 hour | Serves 6**

## Carnitas

1 tablespoon chili powder

1 teaspoon ground coriander

½ cup water

½ teaspoon garlic powder

1 teaspoon fine sea salt

¼ cup fresh lime juice

One 2-pound boneless pork shoulder butt roast, cut into 2-inch cubes

## Rice and Beans

1 cup Minute brand brown rice (see Note)

1½ cups drained cooked black beans, or one 15-ounce can black beans, rinsed and drained

## Pico de Gallo

8 ounces tomatoes (see Note), diced

1 jalapeño chile, seeded and finely diced

1 teaspoon fresh lime juice

¼ cup sliced green onions, white and green parts

3 hearts romaine lettuce, cut into ¼-inch-wide ribbons

Hot sauce (such as Cholula or Tapatío) for serving

½ small yellow onion, diced

1 tablespoon chopped fresh cilantro

Pinch of fine sea salt

2 tablespoons chopped fresh cilantro

2 large avocados, pitted, peeled, and sliced

### To make the carnitas:

1. In a small bowl, combine the chili powder, garlic powder, coriander, and salt and mix well. 2. Pour the water and lime juice into the Instant Pot. Add the pork, arranging the pieces in a single layer. Sprinkle the chili powder mixture evenly over the pork. 3. Secure the lid and set the Pressure Release to Sealing. Select the Meat/Stew setting and set the cooking time for 30 minutes at high pressure. (The pot will take about 10 minutes to come up to pressure before the cooking program begins.) 4. When the cooking program ends, let the pressure release naturally for at least 15 minutes, then move the Pressure Release to Venting to release any remaining steam. Open the pot and, using tongs, transfer the pork to a plate or cutting board. 5. While the pressure is releasing, preheat the oven to 400°F. 6. Wearing heat-resistant mitts, lift out the inner pot and pour the cooking liquid into a fat separator. Pour the defatted cooking liquid into a liquid measuring cup and discard the fat. (Alternatively, use a ladle or large spoon to skim the fat off the surface of the liquid.) Add water as needed to the cooking liquid to total 1 cup (you may have enough without adding water).

### To make the rice and beans:

1. Pour the 1 cup cooking liquid into the Instant Pot and add the rice, making sure it is in an even layer. Place a tall steam rack into the pot. Add the black beans to a 1½-quart stainless-steel bowl and place the bowl on top of the rack. (The bowl should not touch the lid once the pot is closed.) 2. Secure the lid and set the Pressure Release to Sealing. Press the Cancel button to reset the cooking program, then select the Pressure Cook or Manual setting and set the cooking time for 15 minutes at high pressure. (The pot will take about 5 minutes to come to pressure before the cooking program begins.) 3. While the rice and beans are cooking, using two forks, shred the meat into bite-size pieces. Transfer the pork to a sheet pan, spreading it out in an even layer. Place in the oven for 20 minutes, until crispy and browned.

### To make the pico de gallo:

While the carnitas, rice, and beans are cooking, in a medium bowl, combine the tomatoes, onion, jalapeño, cilantro, lime juice, and salt and mix well. Set aside. 1. When the cooking program ends, let the pressure release naturally for 5 minutes, then move the Pressure Release to Venting to release any remaining steam. Open the pot and, wearing heat-resistant mitts, remove the bowl of beans and then the steam rack from the pot. Then remove the inner pot. Add the green onions and cilantro to the rice and, using a fork, fluff the rice and mix in the green onions and cilantro. 2. Divide the rice, beans, carnitas, pico de gallo, lettuce, and avocados evenly among six bowls. Serve warm, with the hot sauce on the side.

**Per Serving**

Calories: 447 | fat: 20g | protein: 31g | carbs: 35g | sugars: 4g | fiber: 9g | sodium: 653mg

# Steak Stroganoff

### Prep time: 15 minutes | Cook time: 30 minutes | Serves 6

1 tablespoon olive oil
½ teaspoon garlic powder
¼ teaspoon paprika
10¾-ounce can reduced-sodium, 98% fat-free cream of mushroom soup
1 envelope sodium-free dried onion soup mix
½ cup fat-free sour cream

2 tablespoons flour
½ teaspoon pepper
1¾-pound boneless beef round steak, trimmed of fat, cut into 1½ × ½-inch strips.
½ cup water
9-ounce jar sliced mushrooms, drained
1 tablespoon minced fresh parsley

1. Place the oil in the Instant Pot and press Sauté. 2. Combine flour, garlic powder, pepper, and paprika in a small bowl. Stir the steak pieces through the flour mixture until they are evenly coated. 3. Lightly brown the steak pieces in the oil in the Instant Pot, about 2 minutes each side. Press Cancel when done. 4. Stir the mushroom soup, water, and onion soup mix then pour over the steak. 5. Secure the lid and set the vent to sealing. Press the Manual button and set for 15 minutes. 6. When cook time is up, let the pressure release naturally for 15 minutes, then release the rest manually. 7. Remove the lid and press Cancel then Sauté. Stir in mushrooms, sour cream, and parsley. Let the sauce come to a boil and cook for about 10–15 minutes.

**Per Serving**
Calories: 248 | fat: 6g | protein: 33g | carbs: 12g | sugars: 2g | fiber: 2g | sodium: 563mg

# Pork Chops Pomodoro

### Prep time: 0 minutes | Cook time: 30 minutes | Serves 6

2 pounds boneless pork loin chops, each about 5⅓ ounces and ½ inch thick
2 tablespoons extra-virgin olive oil
½ cup low-sodium chicken broth or vegetable broth
1 tablespoon capers, drained
2 tablespoons chopped fresh basil or flat-leaf parsley
Lemon wedges for serving

¾ teaspoon fine sea salt
½ teaspoon freshly ground black pepper
2 garlic cloves, chopped
½ teaspoon Italian seasoning
2 cups cherry tomatoes
Spiralized zucchini noodles, cooked cauliflower "rice," or cooked whole-grain pasta for serving

1. Pat the pork chops dry with paper towels, then season them all over with the salt and pepper. 2. Select the Sauté setting on the Instant Pot and heat 1 tablespoon of the oil for 2 minutes. Swirl the oil to coat the bottom of the pot. Using tongs, add half of the pork chops in a single layer and sear for about 3 minutes, until lightly browned on the first side. Flip the chops and sear for about 3 minutes more, until lightly browned on the second side. Transfer the chops to a plate. Repeat with the remaining 1 tablespoon oil and pork chops. 3. Add the garlic to the pot and sauté for about 1 minute, until bubbling but not browned. Stir in the broth, Italian seasoning, and capers, using a wooden spoon to nudge any browned bits from the bottom of the pot and working quickly so not too much liquid evaporates. Using the tongs, transfer the pork chops to the pot. Add the tomatoes in an even layer on top of the chops. 4. Secure the lid and set the Pressure Release to Sealing. Press the Cancel button to reset the cooking program, then select the Pressure Cook or Manual setting and set the cooking time for 10 minutes at high pressure. (The pot will take about 5 minutes to come up to pressure before the cooking program begins.) 5. When the cooking program ends, let the pressure release naturally for at least 10 minutes, then move the Pressure Release to Venting to release any remaining steam. Open the pot and, using the tongs, transfer the pork chops to a serving dish. 6. Spoon the tomatoes and some of the cooking liquid on top of the pork chops. Sprinkle with the basil and serve right away, with zucchini noodles and lemon wedges on the side.

**Per Serving**
Calorie: 265 | fat: 13g | protein: 31g | carbs: 3g | sugars: 2g | fiber: 1g | sodium: 460mg

# Easy Pot Roast and Vegetables

## Prep time: 20 minutes | Cook time: 35 minutes | Serves 6

3–4 pounds chuck roast, trimmed of fat and
cut into serving-sized chunks
2 celery ribs, sliced thin
3 cups water

4 medium potatoes, cubed, unpeeled
4 medium carrots, sliced, or 1 pound baby carrots
1 envelope dry onion soup mix

1. Place the pot roast chunks and vegetables into the Instant Pot along with the potatoes, carrots and celery. 2. Mix together the onion soup mix and water and pour over the contents of the Instant Pot. 3. Secure the lid and make sure the vent is set to sealing. Set the Instant Pot to Manual mode for 35 minutes. Let pressure release naturally when cook time is up.

**Per Serving**
Calorie: 325 | fat: 8g | protein: 35g | carbs: 26g | sugars: 6g | fiber: 4g | sodium: 560mg

# Lamb, Mushroom, and Goat Cheese Burgers

## Prep time: 15 minutes | Cook time: 15 minutes | Serves 4

8 ounces grass-fed ground lamb
¼ teaspoon salt
¼ cup crumbled goat cheese

8 ounces brown mushrooms, finely chopped
¼ teaspoon freshly ground black pepper
1 tablespoon minced fresh basil

1. In a large mixing bowl, combine the lamb, mushrooms, salt, and pepper, and mix well. 2. In a small bowl, mix the goat cheese and basil. 3. Form the lamb mixture into 4 patties, reserving about ½ cup of the mixture in the bowl. In each patty, make an indentation in the center and fill with 1 tablespoon of the goat cheese mixture. Use the reserved meat mixture to close the burgers. Press the meat firmly to hold together. 4. Heat the barbecue or a large skillet over medium-high heat. Add the burgers and cook for 5 to 7 minutes on each side, until cooked through. Serve.

**Per Serving**
Calories: 173 | fat: 13g | protein: 11g | carbs: 3g | sugars: 1g | fiber: 0g | sodium: 154mg

# Zesty Swiss Steak

## Prep time: 35 minutes | Cook time: 35 minutes | Serves 6

3–4 tablespoons flour
½ teaspoon salt
1½ teaspoons dry mustard
1 tablespoon canola oil
1 pound carrots, sliced
⅓ cup water
1½ tablespoons Worcestershire sauce

¼ teaspoon pepper
1½–2 pounds round steak, trimmed of fat
1 cup sliced onions
14½-ounce can whole tomatoes
1 tablespoon brown sugar

1. Combine flour, salt, pepper, and dry mustard. 2. Cut steak in serving pieces. Dredge in flour mixture. 3. Set the Instant Pot to Sauté and add in the oil. Brown the steak pieces on both sides in the oil. Press Cancel. 4. Add onions and carrots into the Instant Pot. 5. Combine the tomatoes, water, brown sugar, and Worcestershire sauce. Pour into the Instant Pot. 6. Secure the lid and make sure the vent is set to sealing. Press Manual and set the time for 35 minutes. 7. When cook time is up, let the pressure release naturally for 15 minutes, then perform a quick release.

**Per Serving**
Calories: 236 | fat: 8g | protein: 23g | carbs: 18g | sugars: 9g | fiber: 3g | sodium: 426mg

# Bavarian Beef

**Prep time: 35 minutes | Cook time: 1 hour 15 minutes | Serves 8**

1 tablespoon canola oil

3 cups sliced carrots

2 large kosher dill pickles, chopped

½ cup dry red wine or beef broth

2 teaspoons coarsely ground black pepper

¼ teaspoon ground cloves

⅓ cup flour

3-pound boneless beef chuck roast, trimmed of fat

3 cups sliced onions

1 cup sliced celery

⅓ cup German-style mustard

2 bay leaves

1 cup water

1. Press Sauté on the Instant Pot and add in the oil. Brown roast on both sides for about 5 minutes. Press Cancel. 2. Add all of the remaining ingredients, except for the flour, to the Instant Pot. 3. Secure the lid and make sure the vent is set to sealing. Press Manual and set the time to 1 hour and 15 minutes. Let the pressure release naturally. 4. Remove meat and vegetables to large platter. Cover to keep warm. 5. Remove 1 cup of the liquid from the Instant Pot and mix with the flour. Press Sauté on the Instant Pot and add the flour/broth mixture back in, whisking. Cook until the broth is smooth and thickened. 6. Serve over noodles or spaetzle.

**Per Serving**

Calories: 251 | fat: 8g | protein: 26g | carbs: 17g | sugars: 7g | fiber: 4g | sodium: 525mg

# "Smothered" Steak

**Prep time: 20 minutes | Cook time: 15 minutes | Serves 6**

1 tablespoon olive oil

⅓ cup flour

1 large onion, sliced

1 green pepper, sliced

4-ounce can mushrooms, drained

10-ounce package frozen French-style green beans

¼ teaspoon pepper

1½-pound chuck, or round, steak, cut into strips, trimmed of fat

14½-ounce can stewed tomatoes

2 tablespoons soy sauce

1. Press Sauté and add the oil to the Instant Pot. 2. Mix together the flour and pepper in a small bowl. Place the steak pieces into the mixture in the bowl and coat each of them well. 3. Lightly brown each of the steak pieces in the Instant Pot, about 2 minutes on each side. Press Cancel when done. 4. Add the remaining ingredients to the Instant Pot and mix together gently. 5. Secure the lid and make sure vent is set to sealing. Press Manual and set for 15 minutes. 6. When cook time is up, let the pressure release naturally for 15 minutes, then perform a quick release.

**Per Serving**

Calories: 386 | fat: 24g | protein: 25g | carbs: 20g | sugars: 4g | fiber: 4g | sodium: 746mg

# Slow-Cooked Simple Lamb and Vegetable Stew

**Prep time: 10 minutes | Cook time: 3 to 10 hours | Serves 6**

1 pound boneless lamb stew meat
1 fennel bulb, trimmed and thinly sliced
1 onion, diced
2 cups low-sodium chicken broth
¼ cup dry red wine (optional)
½ teaspoon salt
Chopped fresh parsley, for garnish

1 pound turnips, peeled and chopped
10 ounces mushrooms, sliced
3 garlic cloves, minced
2 tablespoons tomato paste
1 teaspoon chopped fresh thyme
¼ teaspoon freshly ground black pepper

1. In a slow cooker, combine the lamb, turnips, fennel, mushrooms, onion, garlic, chicken broth, tomato paste, red wine (if using), thyme, salt, and pepper. 2. Cover and cook on high for 3 hours or on low for 6 hours. When the meat is tender and falling apart, garnish with parsley and serve. 3. If you don't have a slow cooker, in a large pot, heat 2 teaspoons of olive oil over medium heat, and sear the lamb on all sides. Remove from the pot and set aside. Add the turnips, fennel, mushrooms, onion, and garlic to the pot, and cook for 3 to 4 minutes until the vegetables begin to soften. Add the chicken broth, tomato paste, red wine (if using), thyme, salt, pepper, and browned lamb. Bring to a boil, then reduce the heat to low. Simmer for 1½ to 2 hours until the meat is tender. Garnish with parsley and serve.

**Per Serving**
Calories: 303 | fat: 7g | protein: 32g | carbs: 27g | sugars: 7g | fiber: 4g | sodium: 310mg

# 30-Minute Garlic Lamb Lollipops

**Prep time: 10 minutes | Cook time: 10 minutes | Serves 4**

2 tablespoons minced garlic
2 tablespoons red wine vinegar
½ teaspoon sea salt
12 to 16 ounces (340 to 454 g) lamb rib chops
Minced fresh rosemary, thyme, or basil, as needed

¼ cup avocado or olive oil
1 tablespoon Italian seasoning
¼ teaspoon black pepper
1 tablespoon avocado or grapeseed oil

1. In a small bowl, combine the garlic, avocado oil, vinegar, Italian seasoning, salt, and black pepper. Whisk to mix the ingredients. 2. Place the lamb rib chops in an airtight container, like a plastic bag or glass storage container. Pour the marinade over the lamb rib chops and let them marinate at room temperature for 10 to 15 minutes. 3. Heat the avocado or grapeseed oil in a large cast-iron skillet over medium-high heat. Gently add the lamb rib chops to the skillet and cook them for 4 minutes. Flip the lamb and cook the meat for another 4 minutes, until it is brown on both sides. 4. Remove the lamb rib chops from the skillet, and let them rest for 10 minutes before serving. Garnish them with the herbs and serve.

**Per Serving**
Calorie: 568 | fat: 54.5g | protein: 19g | carbs: 2g | sugars: 0g | fiber: 0g | sodium: 361mg

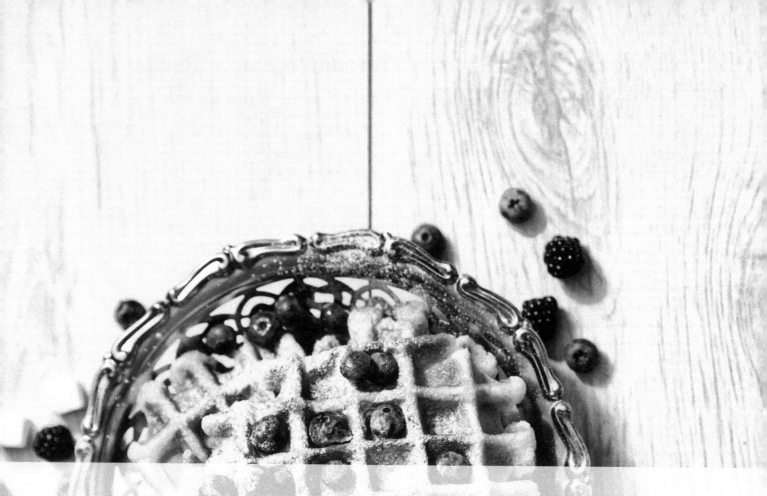
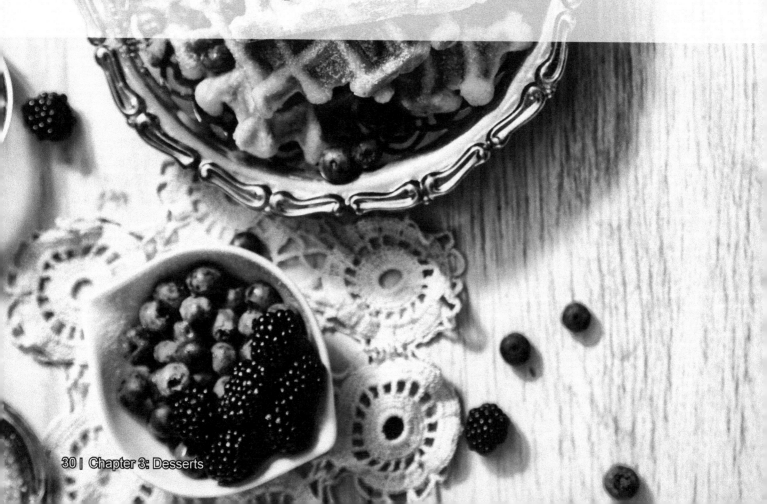

# Chapter 3 Desserts

# Peanut Butter Fudge Brownies

## Prep time: 5 minutes | Cook time: 15 minutes | Makes 12 brownies

Cooking oil spray, as needed
½ cup almond flour
¼ cup cooking oil of choice
¼ teaspoon baking soda
¼ teaspoon sea salt
⅓ cup unsweetened cocoa powder
¼ cup dairy-free dark chocolate chips

1 cup gluten-free rolled oats
1 cup canned low-sodium black beans, drained and rinsed
1½ teaspoon pure vanilla extract
1 teaspoon baking powder
1 teaspoon ground cinnamon
½ cup pure maple syrup
2 tablespoons all-natural peanut butter (see Tip)

1. Preheat the oven to 350°F (177°C). Spray an 8 x 8–inch (20 x 20–cm) baking pan with the cooking oil spray. 2. In a food processor, combine the oats, almond flour, beans, oil, vanilla, baking soda, baking powder, sea salt, cinnamon, cocoa powder, and maple syrup. Process the ingredients for about 1 minute, until the batter is smooth. You may need to stop the food processor once and scrape down the sides. 3. Carefully remove the food processor's blade and stir in the chocolate chips by hand. 4. Spread the batter into the prepared baking pan. Drizzle the peanut butter over the top of the batter. 5. Bake the brownies for 15 minutes, until a toothpick inserted into the center comes out clean. Let the brownies cool completely in the pan on a wire rack.

**Per Serving**

Calorie: 170 | fat: 10g | protein: 3g | carbs: 19g | sugars: 11g | fiber: 2g | sodium: 52mg

# Cherry Delight

## Prep time: 20 minutes | Cook time: 50 minutes | Serves 12

20-ounce can cherry pie filling, light
¼ cup light, soft tub margarine, melted
1 cup water

½ package yellow cake mix
⅓ cup walnuts, optional

1. Grease a 7" springform pan then pour the pie filing inside. 2. Combine dry cake mix and margarine (mixture will be crumbly) in a bowl. Sprinkle over filling. Sprinkle with walnuts. 3. Cover the pan with foil. 4. Place the trivet into your Instant Pot and pour in 1 cup of water. Place a foil sling on top of the trivet, then place the springform pan on top. 5. Secure the lid and make sure lid is set to sealing. Press Steam and set for 50 minutes. 6. When cook time is up, release the pressure manually, then carefully remove the springform pan by using hot pads to lift the pan up by the foil sling. Place on a cooling rack for 1–2 hours.

**Per Serving**

Calories: 137| fat: 4g | protein: 1g | carbs: 26g | sugars: 19g | fiber: 1g | sodium: 174mg

# Frozen Mocha Milkshake

## Prep time: 5 minutes | Cook time: 0 minutes | Serves 1

1 cup unsweetened vanilla almond milk
2 teaspoons instant espresso powder
½ medium avocado, peeled and pitted
1 teaspoon pure vanilla extract

3 tablespoons unsweetened cocoa powder
1½ cups crushed ice
1 tablespoon pure maple syrup

1. In a blender, combine the almond milk, cocoa powder, espresso powder, ice, avocado, maple syrup, and vanilla. Blend the ingredients on high speed for 60 seconds, until the milkshake is smooth.

**Per Serving**

Calorie: 307 | fat: 20g | protein: 6g | carbs: 33g | sugars: 13g | fiber: 13g | sodium: 173mg

# 5-Ingredient Chunky Cherry and Peanut Butter Cookies

## Prep time: 5 minutes | Cook time: 10 to 12 minutes | Makes 12 cookies

1 cup all-natural peanut butter
1 large egg, beaten
½ cup dried cherries

¼ cup pure maple syrup
1 cup gluten-free rolled or quick oats

1. Preheat the oven to 350°F (177°C). Line a large baking sheet with parchment paper. 2. In a large bowl, whisk together the peanut butter, maple syrup, and egg. Add the oats and cherries, and mix until the ingredients are combined. 3. Chill the dough for 10 to 15 minutes. 4. Use a cookie scoop to scoop balls of the dough onto the prepared baking sheet. 5. Using a fork, gently flatten the dough balls into your desired shape (the cookies will not change shape much during baking). Bake the cookies for 10 to 12 minutes, until they are lightly golden on top. 6. Remove the cookies from the oven and let them cool for 5 minutes before transferring them to a wire rack.
**Per Serving**
Calorie: 198 | fat: 12g | protein: 7g | carbs: 19g | sugars: 11g | fiber: 3g | sodium: 13mg

# Strawberry Chia Pudding

## Prep time: 5 minutes | Cook time: 0 minutes | Serves 2

1½ cups frozen whole strawberries
1 tablespoon coconut nectar or pure maple syrup
Pinch of sea salt

3 tablespoons white chia seeds
1 teaspoon lemon juice
½ cup + 2–3 tablespoons plain low-fat nondairy milk

1. In a blender, combine the strawberries, chia seeds, nectar or syrup, lemon juice, salt, and ½ cup plus 2 tablespoons of the milk. Puree until the seeds are fully pulverized and the pudding begins to thicken. (It will thicken more as it cools.) Add the extra 1 tablespoon milk if needed to blend. Transfer the mixture to a large bowl or dish and refrigerate until chilled, about an hour or more. (It will thicken more with chilling, but really can be eaten right away.)
**Per Serving**
Calorie: 185 | fat: 5g | protein: 4g | carbs: 33g | sugars: 16g | fiber: 9g | sodium: 182mg

# Mixed-Berry Snack Cake

## Prep time: 15 minutes | Cook time: 28 to 33 minutes | Serves 8

¼ cup low-fat granola
⅓ cup packed brown sugar
1 teaspoon vanilla
1 cup whole wheat flour
½ teaspoon ground cinnamon
1 cup mixed fresh berries (such as blueberries, raspberries and blackberries)

½ cup buttermilk
2 tablespoons canola oil
1 egg
½ teaspoon baking soda
⅛ teaspoon salt

1. Heat oven to 350°F. Spray 8- or 9-inch round pan with cooking spray. Place granola in resealable food-storage plastic bag; seal bag and slightly crush with rolling pin or meat mallet. Set aside. 2. In large bowl, stir buttermilk, brown sugar, oil, vanilla and egg until smooth. Stir in flour, baking soda, cinnamon and salt just until moistened. Gently fold in half of the berries. Spoon into pan. Sprinkle with remaining berries and the granola. 3. Bake 28 to 33 minutes or until golden brown and top springs back when touched in center. Cool in pan on cooling rack 10 minutes. Serve warm.
**Per Serving**
Calorie: 160 | fat: 5g | protein: 3g | carbs: 26g | sugars: 12g | fiber: 1g | sodium: 140mg

# Ginger Cake with Caramel-Apple Topping

## Prep time: 15 minutes | Cook time: 38 to 43 minutes | Serves 15

2 cups harvest peach or vanilla fat-free yogurt
1¼ cups whole wheat flour
¼ cup sugar
1 teaspoon ground cinnamon
½ teaspoon salt
⅓ cup canola oil
1 medium tart apple, chopped

½ cup caramel fat-free topping
1 cup all-purpose flour
1 teaspoon baking soda
1 teaspoon ground ginger
½ cup molasses
1 egg
Lemon juice

1. Heat oven to 350°F. Grease and flour 9-inch square pan. In medium bowl, mix ¾ cup of the yogurt and the caramel topping; cover and refrigerate until serving time. 2. In large bowl, beat remaining 1¼ cups yogurt and all remaining ingredients except apple and lemon juice with electric mixer on low speed 45 seconds, scraping bowl constantly. Beat on medium speed 1 minute, scraping bowl occasionally, until well blended. Stir in half of the chopped apple. Pour batter into pan. Sprinkle lemon juice over remaining apple; cover and refrigerate until serving time. 3. Bake 38 to 43 minutes or until toothpick inserted in center comes out clean. Cool slightly. Serve with topping mixture and remaining chopped apple.

**Per Serving**

Calorie: 230 | fat: 6g | protein: 3g | carbs: 40g | sugars: 21g | fiber: 2g | sodium: 220mg

# Baked Berry Cups with Crispy Cinnamon Wedges

## Prep time: 25 minutes | Cook time: 30 minutes | Serves 4

2 teaspoons sugar
Butter-flavor cooking spray
¼ cup sugar
1 teaspoon grated orange peel, if desired
1½ cups fresh raspberries

¾ teaspoon ground cinnamon
1 balanced carb whole wheat tortilla (6 inch)
2 tablespoons white whole wheat flour
1½ cups fresh blueberries
About 1 cup fat-free whipped cream topping
(from aerosol can)

1. Heat oven to 375°F. In sandwich-size resealable food-storage plastic bag, combine 2 teaspoons sugar and ½ teaspoon of the cinnamon. Using cooking spray, spray both sides of tortilla, about 3 seconds per side; cut tortilla into 8 wedges. In bag with cinnamon-sugar, add wedges; seal bag. Shake to coat wedges evenly. 2. On ungreased cookie sheet, spread out wedges. Bake 7 to 9 minutes, turning once, until just beginning to crisp (wedges will continue to crisp while cooling). Cool about 15 minutes. 3. Meanwhile, spray 4 (6-ounce) custard cups or ramekins with cooking spray; place cups on another cookie sheet. In small bowl, stir ¼ cup sugar, the flour, orange peel and remaining ¼ teaspoon cinnamon until blended. In medium bowl, gently toss berries with sugar mixture; divide evenly among custard cups. 4. Bake 15 minutes; stir gently. Bake 5 to 7 minutes longer or until liquid is bubbling around edges. Cool at least 15 minutes. 5 To serve, top each cup with about ¼ cup whipped cream topping; serve tortilla wedges with berry cups. Serve warm.

**Per Serving**

Calorie: 180 | fat: 2g | protein: 3g | carbs: 37g | sugars: 25g | fiber: 7g | sodium: 60mg

# Raspberry Nice Cream

## Prep time: 5 minutes | Cook time: 0 minutes | Serves 3

| | |
|---|---|
| 2 cups frozen, sliced, overripe bananas | 2 cups frozen or fresh raspberries |
| Pinch of sea salt | 1–2 tablespoons coconut nectar or |
| | 1–1½ tablespoons pure maple syrup |

1. In a food processor or high-speed blender, combine the bananas, raspberries, salt, and 1 tablespoon of the nectar or syrup. Puree until smooth. Taste, and add the remaining nectar or syrup, if desired. Serve immediately, if you like a soft-serve consistency, or transfer to an airtight container and freeze for an hour or more, if you like a firmer texture.

**Per Serving**

Calorie: 193| fat: 1g | protein: 3g | carbs: 47g | sugars: 24g | fiber: 13g | sodium: 101mg

# Oatmeal Chippers

## Prep time: 10 minutes | Cook time: 11 minutes | Makes 20 chippers

| | |
|---|---|
| 3–3½ tablespoons almond butter | ¼ cup pure maple syrup |
| (or tigernut butter, for nut-free) | ¼ cup brown rice syrup |
| 2 teaspoons pure vanilla extract | 1⅓ cups oat flour |
| 1 cup + 2 tablespoons rolled oats | 1½ teaspoons baking powder |
| ½ teaspoon cinnamon | ¼ teaspoon sea salt |
| 2–3 tablespoons sugar-free nondairy chocolate chips | |

1. Preheat the oven to 350°F. Line a baking sheet with parchment paper. 2. In the bowl of a mixer, combine the almond butter, maple syrup, brown rice syrup, and vanilla. Using the paddle attachment, mix on low speed for a couple of minutes, until creamy. Turn off the mixer and add the flour, oats, baking powder, cinnamon, salt, and chocolate chips. Mix on low speed until incorporated. Place 1½-tablespoon mounds on the prepared baking sheet, spacing them 1" to 2" apart, and flatten slightly. Bake for 11 minutes, or until just set to the touch. Remove from the oven, let cool on the pan for just a minute, and then transfer the cookies to a cooling rack.

**Per Serving**

Calorie: 90 | fat: 2g | protein: 2g | carbs: 16g | sugars: 4g | fiber: 2g | sodium: 75mg

# Grilled Peach and Coconut Yogurt Bowls

## Prep time: 5 minutes | Cook time: 10 minutes | Serves 4

| | |
|---|---|
| 2 peaches, halved and pitted | ½ cup plain nonfat Greek yogurt |
| 1 teaspoon pure vanilla extract | ¼ cup unsweetened dried coconut flakes |
| 2 tablespoons unsalted pistachios, shelled and broken into pieces | |

1. Preheat the broiler to high. Arrange the rack in the closest position to the broiler. 2. In a shallow pan, arrange the peach halves, cut-side up. Broil for 6 to 8 minutes until browned, tender, and hot. 3. In a small bowl, mix the yogurt and vanilla. 4. Spoon the yogurt into the cavity of each peach half. 5. Sprinkle 1 tablespoon of coconut flakes and 1½ teaspoons of pistachios over each peach half. Serve warm.

**Per Serving**

Calories: 102 | fat: 5g | protein: 5g | carbs: 11g | sugars: 8g | fiber: 2g | sodium: 12mg

# Chocolate Baked Bananas

**Prep time: 10 minutes | Cook time: 8 to 10 minutes | Serves 5**

4–5 large ripe bananas, sliced lengthwise
1 tablespoon cocoa powder
2 tablespoons nondairy chocolate chips (for finishing) or pumpkin seeds (for finishing)

2 tablespoons coconut nectar or pure maple syrup
Couple pinches sea salt
1 tablespoon chopped pecans, walnuts, almonds, or

1. Line a baking sheet with parchment paper and preheat oven to 450°F. Place bananas on the parchment. In a bowl, mix the coconut nectar or maple syrup with the cocoa powder and salt. Stir well to fully combine. Drizzle the chocolate mixture over the bananas. Bake for 8 to 10 minutes, until bananas are softened and caramelized. Sprinkle on chocolate chips and nuts, and serve.

**Per Serving**
Calorie: 146 | fat: 3g | protein: 2g | carbs: 34g | sugars: 18g | fiber: 4g | sodium: 119mg

# Quick Yummy Peaches

**Prep time: 20 minutes | Cook time: 20 minutes | Serves 8**

⅓ cup buttermilk baking mix
¼ cup brown sugar
1 teaspoon cinnamon
½ cup peach juice or water

⅔ cup dry quick oats
Brown sugar substitute to equal 2 tablespoons sugar
4 cups sliced peaches, canned or fresh
1 cup water

1. Mix together baking mix, oats, brown sugar, brown sugar substitute, and cinnamon. Mix in the peaches and peach juice. 2. Pour mixture into a 1.6-quart baking dish. Cover with foil. 3. Place the trivet into your Instant Pot and pour in 1 cup of water. Place a foil sling on top of the trivet, then place the baking dish on top. 4. Secure the lid and make sure lid is set to sealing. Press Manual and set for 10 minutes. 5. When cook time is up, let the pressure release naturally for 10 minutes, then release any remaining pressure manually. Carefully remove the baking dish by using hot pads to lift the foil sling. Uncover and let cool for about 20–30 minutes.

**Per Serving**
Calories: 131 | fat: 1g | protein: 2g | carbs: 29g | sugars: 20g | fiber: 3g | sodium: 76mg

# Greek Yogurt Strawberry Pops

**Prep time: 5 minutes | Cook time: 0 minutes | Serves 6**

2 ripe bananas, peeled, cut into ½-inch pieces, and frozen
½ cup plain 2 percent Greek yogurt
1 cup chopped fresh strawberries

1. In a food processor, combine the bananas and yogurt and process at high speed for 2 minutes, until mostly smooth (it's okay if a few small chunks remain). Scrape down the sides of the bowl, add the strawberries, and process for 1 minute, until smooth. 2. Divide the mixture evenly among six ice-pop molds. Tap each mold on a countertop a few times to get rid of any air pockets, then place an ice-pop stick into each mold and transfer the molds to the freezer. Freeze for at least 4 hours, or until frozen solid. 3. To unmold each ice pop, run it under cold running water for 5 seconds, taking care not to get water inside the mold, then remove the ice pop from the mold. Eat the ice pops right away or store in a ziplock plastic freezer bag in the freezer for up to 2 months.

**Per Serving**
Calories: 57 | fat: 1g | protein: 3g | carbs: 12g | sugars: 6g | fiber: 2g | sodium: 8mg

# Strawberry Cream Cheese Crepes

## Prep time: 10 minutes | Cook time: 10 minutes | Serves 4

| | |
|---|---|
| ½ cup old-fashioned oats | 1 cup unsweetened plain almond milk |
| 1 egg | 3 teaspoons honey, divided |
| Nonstick cooking spray | 2 ounces low-fat cream cheese |
| ¼ cup low-fat cottage cheese | 2 cups sliced strawberries |

1. In a blender jar, process the oats until they resemble flour. Add the almond milk, egg, and 1½ teaspoons honey, and process until smooth. 2. Heat a large skillet over medium heat. Spray with nonstick cooking spray to coat. 3. Add ¼ cup of oat batter to the pan and quickly swirl around to coat the bottom of the pan and let cook for 2 to 3 minutes. When the edges begin to turn brown, flip the crepe with a spatula and cook until lightly browned and firm, about 1 minute. Transfer to a plate. Continue with the remaining batter, spraying the skillet with nonstick cooking spray before adding more batter. Set the cooked crepes aside, loosely covered with aluminum foil, while you make the filling. 4. Clean the blender jar, then combine the cream cheese, cottage cheese, and remaining 1½ teaspoons honey, and process until smooth. 5. Fill each crepe with 2 tablespoons of the cream cheese mixture, topped with ¼ cup of strawberries. Serve.

**Per Serving**

Calories: 149 | fat: 6g | protein: 6g | carbs: 20g | sugars: 10g | fiber: 3g | sodium: 177mg

# Chewy Chocolate-Oat Bars

## Prep time: 20 minutes | Cook time: 30 minutes | Makes 16 bars

| | |
|---|---|
| ¾ cup semisweet chocolate chips | ⅓ cup fat-free sweetened condensed milk |
| 1 cup whole wheat flour | (from 14-ounce can) |
| ½ cup quick-cooking oats | ½ teaspoon baking powder |
| ½ teaspoon baking soda | ¼ teaspoon salt |
| ¼ cup fat-free egg product or 1 egg | ¾ cup packed brown sugar |
| ¼ cup canola oil | 1 teaspoon vanilla |
| 2 tablespoons quick-cooking oats | 2 teaspoons butter or margarine, softened |

1. Heat oven to 350°F. Spray 8-inch or 9-inch square pan with cooking spray. 2. In 1-quart saucepan, heat chocolate chips and milk over low heat, stirring frequently, until chocolate is melted and mixture is smooth. Remove from heat. 3. In large bowl, mix flour, ½ cup oats, the baking powder, baking soda and salt; set aside. In medium bowl, stir egg product, brown sugar, oil and vanilla with fork until smooth. Stir into flour mixture until blended. Reserve ½ cup dough in small bowl for topping. 4. Pat remaining dough in pan (if dough is sticky, spray fingers with cooking spray or dust with flour). Spread chocolate mixture over dough. Add 2 tablespoons oats and the butter to reserved ½ cup dough; mix with pastry blender or fork until well mixed. Place small pieces of mixture evenly over chocolate mixture. 5 Bake 20 to 25 minutes or until top is golden and firm. Cool completely, about 1 hour 30 minutes. For bars, cut into 4 rows by 4 rows.

**Per Serving**

Calorie: 180 | fat: 7g | protein: 3g | carbs: 27g | sugars: 18g | fiber: 1g | sodium: 115mg

# Cream Cheese Swirl Brownies

## Prep time: 10 minutes | Cook time: 20 minutes | Serves 12

2 eggs
¼ cup coconut oil, melted
¼ cup unsweetened cocoa powder
¼ teaspoon salt
2 tablespoons low-fat cream cheese

¼ cup unsweetened applesauce
3 tablespoons pure maple syrup, divided
¼ cup coconut flour
1 teaspoon baking powder

1. Preheat the oven to 350°F. Grease an 8-by-8-inch baking dish. 2. In a large mixing bowl, beat the eggs with the applesauce, coconut oil, and 2 tablespoons of maple syrup. 3. Stir in the cocoa powder and coconut flour, and mix well. Sprinkle the salt and baking powder evenly over the surface and mix well to incorporate. Transfer the mixture to the prepared baking dish. 4. In a small, microwave-safe bowl, microwave the cream cheese for 10 to 20 seconds until softened. Add the remaining 1 tablespoon of maple syrup and mix to combine. 5. Drop the cream cheese onto the batter, and use a toothpick or chopstick to swirl it on the surface. Bake for 20 minutes, until a toothpick inserted in the center comes out clean. Cool and cut into 12 squares. 6. Store refrigerated in a covered container for up to 5 days.

**Per Serving**
Calories: 84 | fat: 6g | protein: 2g | carbs: 6g | sugars: 4g | fiber: 2g | sodium: 93mg

# Fudgy Walnut Brownies

## Prep time: 10 minutes | Cook time: 1 hour | Serves 12

¾ cup walnut halves and pieces
4 large eggs
1½ teaspoons vanilla extract
¼ teaspoon fine sea salt
¾ cup natural cocoa powder

½ cup unsalted butter, melted and cooled
1½ teaspoons instant coffee crystals
1 cup Lakanto Monkfruit Sweetener Golden
¾ cup almond flour
¾ cup stevia-sweetened chocolate chips

1. In a dry small skillet over medium heat, toast the walnuts, stirring often, for about 5 minutes, until golden. Transfer the walnuts to a bowl to cool. 2. Pour 1 cup water into the Instant Pot. Line the base of a 7 by 3-inch round cake pan with a circle of parchment paper. Butter the sides of the pan and the parchment or coat with nonstick cooking spray. 3. Pour the butter into a medium bowl. One at a time, whisk in the eggs, then whisk in the coffee crystals, vanilla, sweetener, and salt. Finally, whisk in the flour and cocoa powder just until combined. Using a rubber spatula, fold in the chocolate chips and walnuts. 4. Transfer the batter to the prepared pan and, using the spatula, spread it in an even layer. Cover the pan tightly with aluminum foil. Place the pan on a long-handled silicone steam rack, then, holding the handles of the steam rack, lower it into the Instant Pot. 5. Secure the lid and set the Pressure Release to Sealing. Select the Cake, Pressure Cook, or Manual setting and set the cooking time for 45 minutes at high pressure. (The pot will take about 10 minutes to come up to pressure before the cooking program begins.) 6. When the cooking program ends, let the pressure release naturally for 10 minutes, then move the Pressure Release to Venting to release any remaining steam. Open the pot and, wearing heat-resistant mitts, grasp the handles of the steam rack and lift it out of the pot. Uncover the pan, taking care not to get burned by the steam or to drip condensation onto the brownies. Let the brownies cool in the pan on a cooling rack for about 2 hours, to room temperature. 7. Run a butter knife around the edge of the pan to make sure the brownies are not sticking to the pan sides. Invert the brownies onto the rack, lift off the pan, and peel off the parchment paper. Invert the brownies onto a serving plate and cut into twelve wedges. The brownies will keep, stored in an airtight container in the refrigerator for up to 5 days, or in the freezer for up to 4 months.

**Per Serving**
Calories: 199 | fat: 19g | protein: 5g | carbs: 26g | sugars: 10g | fiber: 20g | sodium: 56mg

# Pomegranate–Tequila Sunrise Jelly Shots

## Prep time: 30 minutes | Cook time: 10 minutes | Serves 12

¾ cup pulp-free orange juice
6 tablespoons silver or gold tequila
¼ cup sugar
Whole orange slices or orange slice wedges

2 envelopes unflavored gelatin
½ cup 100% pomegranate juice
¼ cup water

1. Lightly spray 12 (2-ounce) shot glasses with cooking spray; gently wipe any excess with paper towel. In 1-quart saucepan, pour orange juice; sprinkle 1 envelope gelatin evenly over juice to soften. Heat over low heat, stirring constantly, until gelatin is completely dissolved; remove from heat. Stir in tequila. Divide orange juice mixture evenly among shot glasses (about 2 tablespoons per glass). In 9-inch square pan, place shot glasses. Refrigerate 30 minutes or until almost set. 2. Meanwhile, in same saucepan, combine pomegranate juice, sugar and water. Sprinkle remaining 1 envelope gelatin evenly over juice to soften. Heat over low heat, stirring constantly, until gelatin is completely dissolved; remove from heat. 3. Remove shot glasses from refrigerator (orange layer should appear mostly set). Pour pomegranate mixture evenly over top of orange layer in glasses (about 4 teaspoons per glass). Refrigerate at least 3 hours until completely chilled and firm. 4. Just before serving, dip a table knife in hot water; slide knife along inside edge of shot glass to loosen. Shake jelly shot out of glass onto plate; repeat with remaining jelly shots. Serve each jelly shot on top of whole orange slice or serve jelly shots with orange slice wedges.

**Per Serving**
Calorie: 60 | fat: 0g | protein: 1g | carbs: 9g | sugars: 9g | fiber: 0g | sodium: 0mg

# Almond Butter Blondies

## Prep time: 10 minutes | Cook time: 20 minutes | Serves 8

½ cup creamy natural almond butter, at room temperature
¾ cup Lakanto Monkfruit Sweetener Golden
½ teaspoon fine sea salt
¾ cup stevia-sweetened chocolate chips

4 large eggs
1 teaspoon pure vanilla extract
1¼ cups almond flour

1. Pour 1 cup water into the Instant Pot. Line the base of a 7 by 3-inch round cake pan with a circle of parchment paper. Butter the sides of the pan and the parchment or coat with nonstick cooking spray. 2. Put the almond butter into a medium bowl. One at a time, whisk the eggs into the almond butter, then whisk in the sweetener, vanilla, and salt. Stir in the flour just until it is fully incorporated, followed by the chocolate chips. 3. Transfer the batter to the prepared pan and, using a rubber spatula, spread it in an even layer. Cover the pan tightly with aluminum foil. Place the pan on a long-handled silicone steam rack, then, holding the handles of the steam rack, lower it into the Instant Pot. 4. Secure the lid and set the Pressure Release to Sealing. Select the Cake, Pressure Cook, or Manual setting and set the cooking time for 40 minutes at high pressure. (The pot will take about 10 minutes to come up to pressure before the cooking program begins.) 5. When the cooking program ends, let the pressure release naturally for 10 minutes, then move the Pressure Release to Venting to release any remaining steam. Open the pot and, wearing heat-resistant mitts, grasp the handles of the steam rack and lift it out of the pot. Uncover the pan, taking care not to get burned by the steam or to drip condensation onto the blondies. Let the blondies cool in the pan on a cooling rack for about 5 minutes. 6. Run a butter knife around the edge of pan to make sure the blondies are not sticking to the pan sides. Invert the blondies onto the rack, lift off the pan, and peel off the parchment paper. Let cool for 15 minutes, then invert the blondies onto a serving plate and cut into eight wedges. The blondies will keep, stored in an airtight container in the refrigerator for up to 5 days, or in the freezer for up to 4 months.

**Per Serving**
Calories: 211 | fat: 17g | protein: 8g | carbs: 20g | sugars: 10g | fiber: 17g | sodium: 186mg

# Oatmeal Cookies

## Prep time: 5 minutes | Cook time: 15 minutes | Serves 16

¾ cup almond flour
¼ cup shredded unsweetened coconut
1 teaspoon ground cinnamon
¼ cup unsweetened applesauce
1 tablespoon pure maple syrup

¾ cup old-fashioned oats
1 teaspoon baking powder
¼ teaspoon salt
1 large egg
2 tablespoons coconut oil, melted

1. Preheat the oven to 350°F. 2. In a medium mixing bowl, combine the almond flour, oats, coconut, baking powder, cinnamon, and salt, and mix well. 3. In another medium bowl, combine the applesauce, egg, maple syrup, and coconut oil, and mix. Stir the wet mixture into the dry mixture. 4. Form the dough into balls a little bigger than a tablespoon and place on a baking sheet, leaving at least 1 inch between them. Bake for 12 minutes until the cookies are just browned. Remove from the oven and let cool for 5 minutes. 5. Using a spatula, remove the cookies and cool on a rack.

**Per Serving**
Calorie: 76 | fat: 6g | protein: 2g | carbs: 5g | sugars: 1g | fiber: 1g | sodium: 57mg

# Blender Banana Snack Cake

## Prep time: 5 minutes | Cook time: 30 to 32 minutes | Serves 9

¼ cup coconut nectar or pure maple syrup
2 teaspoons vanilla
½ teaspoon nutmeg
3½ cups sliced, well-ripened bananas
½ cup rolled oats

¼ cup water
1 teaspoon cinnamon
¼ teaspoon sea salt
1 cup whole grain spelt flour
2 teaspoons baking powder

1. Preheat the oven to 350°F. Lightly coat an 8" x 8" pan with cooking spray and line the bottom of the pan with parchment paper. 2. In a blender, combine the nectar or syrup, water, vanilla, cinnamon, nutmeg, salt, and 3 cups of the sliced bananas. Puree until smooth. Add the flour, oats, baking powder, and the remaining ½ cup of bananas. Pulse a couple of times, until just combined. (Don't puree; you don't want to overwork the flour.) Transfer the mixture into the baking dish, using a spatula to scrape down the sides of the bowl. Bake for 30 to 32 minutes, until fully set. (Insert a toothpick in the center and see if it comes out clean.) Transfer the cake pan to a cooling rack. Let cool completely before cutting.

**Per Serving**
Calorie: 141 | fat: 1g | protein: 3g | carbs: 32g | sugars: 14g | fiber: 4g | sodium: 177mg

# Dulce de Leche Fillo Cups

## Prep time: 15 minutes | Cook time: 0 minutes | Serves 15

2 ounces ⅓-less-fat cream cheese (Neufchâtel), softened
1 tablespoon reduced-fat sour cream
⅓ cup sliced fresh strawberries

2 tablespoons dulce de leche (caramel) syrup
1 package frozen mini fillo shells (15 shells)
2 tablespoons diced mango

1 In medium bowl, beat cream cheese with electric mixer on low speed until creamy. Beat in dulce de leche syrup and sour cream until blended. 2 Spoon cream cheese mixture into each fillo shell. Top each with strawberries and mango.

**Per Serving**
Calorie: 40 | fat: 2g | protein: 0g | carbs: 4g | sugars: 2g | fiber: 0g | sodium: 35mg

# Chewy Barley-Nut Cookies

## Prep time: 45 minutes | Cook time: 10 to 14 minutes | Makes 2 dozen cookies

⅓ cup canola oil
¼ cup packed brown sugar
1 teaspoon vanilla
2 cups rolled barley flakes or 2 cups plus
2 tablespoons old-fashioned oats
½ teaspoon salt
⅓ cup "heart-healthy" mixed nuts (peanuts, almonds, pistachios, pecans, hazelnuts)

½ cup granulated sugar
¼ cup reduced-fat mayonnaise or salad dressing
1 egg
¾ cup whole wheat flour
½ teaspoon baking soda
¼ teaspoon ground cinnamon

1. Heat oven to 350°F. Spray cookie sheet with cooking spray. 2 In medium bowl, mix oil, sugars, mayonnaise, vanilla and egg with spoon. Stir in barley, flour, baking soda, salt and cinnamon. Stir in nuts. 3. Drop dough by rounded tablespoonfuls 2. inches apart onto cookie sheet. 4. Bake 10 to 14 minutes or until edges are golden brown. Cool 2 minutes; transfer from cookie sheet to cooling rack.

**Per Serving**
Calorie: 150 | fat: 5g | protein: 2g | carbs: 23g | sugars: 7g | fiber: 3g | sodium: 110mg

# Mixed-Berry Cream Tart

## Prep time: 20 minutes | Cook time: 0 minutes | Serves 8

2 cups sliced fresh strawberries
1 box (4-serving size) sugar-free strawberry gelatin
1 package (8 ounces) fat-free cream cheese
¼ cup sugar
1 cup fresh blueberries
Fat-free whipped topping, if desired

½ cup boiling water
3 pouches (1.5 ounces each) roasted almond crunchy granola bars (from 8.9-ounce box)
¼ teaspoon almond extract
1 cup fresh raspberries

1. In small bowl, crush 1 cup of the strawberries with pastry blender or fork. Reserve remaining 1 cup strawberries. 2. In medium bowl, pour boiling water over gelatin; stir about 2 minutes or until gelatin is completely dissolved. Stir crushed strawberries into gelatin. Refrigerate 20 minutes. 3. Meanwhile, leaving granola bars in pouches, crush granola bars with rolling pin. Sprinkle crushed granola in bottom of 9-inch ungreased glass pie plate, pushing crumbs up side of plate to make crust. 4. In small bowl, beat cream cheese, sugar and almond extract with electric mixer on medium-high speed until smooth. Drop by spoonfuls over crushed granola; gently spread to cover bottom of crust. 5. Gently fold blueberries, raspberries and remaining 1 cup strawberries into gelatin mixture. Spoon over cream cheese mixture. Refrigerate about 3 hours or until firm. Serve topped with whipped topping.

**Per Serving**
Calorie: 170 | fat: 3g | protein: 8g | carbs: 27g | sugars: 17g | fiber: 3g | sodium: 340mg

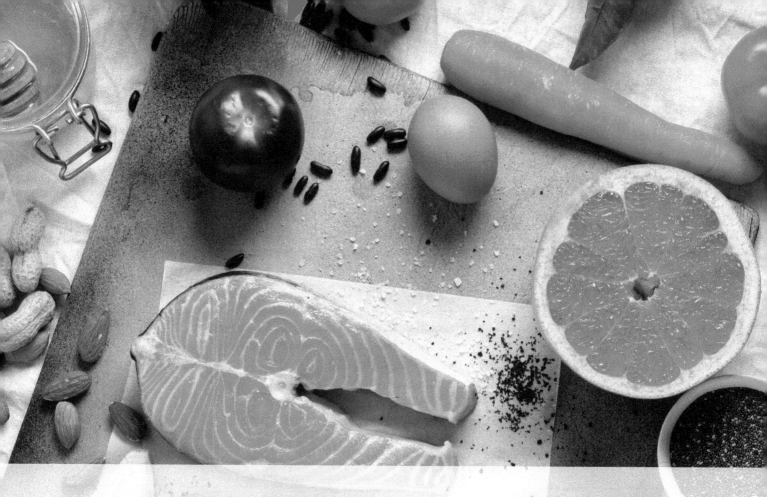

# Chapter 4    Fish and Seafood

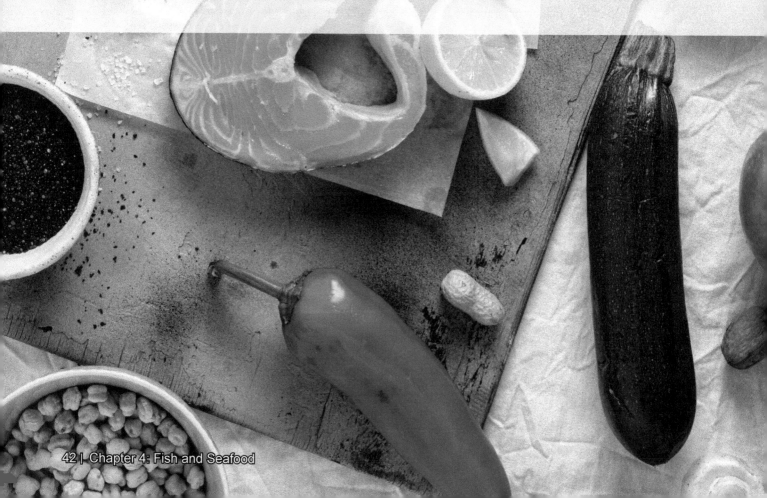

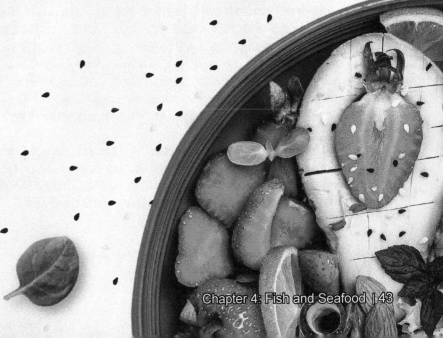

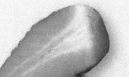

# Peppercorn-Crusted Baked Salmon

## Prep time: 5 minutes | Cook time: 20 minutes | Serves 4

Nonstick cooking spray
¼ teaspoon salt
¼ teaspoon dried thyme

½ teaspoon freshly ground black pepper
Zest and juice of ½ lemon
1 pound salmon fillet

1. Preheat the oven to 425°F. Spray a baking sheet with nonstick cooking spray. 2. In a small bowl, combine the pepper, salt, lemon zest and juice, and thyme. Stir to combine. 3. Place the salmon on the prepared baking sheet, skin-side down. Spread the seasoning mixture evenly over the fillet. 4. Bake for 15 to 20 minutes, depending on the thickness of the fillet, until the flesh flakes easily.

**Per Serving**

Calories: 163 | fat: 7g | protein: 23g | carbs: 1g | sugars: 0g | fiber: 0g | sodium: 167mg

# Shrimp Louie Salad with Thousand Island Dressing

## Prep time: 5 minutes | Cook time: 20 minutes | Serves 4

2 cups water
1 pound medium shrimp, peeled and deveined
Thousand island Dressing
¼ cup mayonnaise
1 teaspoon Worcestershire sauce
Freshly ground black pepper
2 hearts romaine lettuce or 1 head iceberg lettuce, shredded
1 cup cherry tomatoes, sliced

1½ teaspoons fine sea salt
4 large eggs
¼ cup no-sugar-added ketchup
1 tablespoon fresh lemon juice
⅛ teaspoon cayenne pepper
2 green onions, white and green parts, sliced thinly
1 English cucumber, sliced
8 radishes, sliced
1 large avocado, pitted, peeled, and sliced

Combine the water and salt in the Instant Pot and stir to dissolve the salt. 2. Secure the lid and set the Pressure Release to Sealing. Select the Steam setting and set the cooking time for 0 (zero) minutes at low pressure. (The pot will take about 10 minutes to come up to pressure before the cooking program begins.) 3. Meanwhile, prepare an ice bath. 4. When the cooking program ends, perform a quick release by moving the Pressure Release to Venting. Open the pot and stir in the shrimp, using a wooden spoon to nudge them all down into the water. Cover the pot and leave the shrimp for 2 minutes on the Keep Warm setting. The shrimp will gently poach and cook through. Uncover the pot and, wearing heat-resistant mitts, lift out the inner pot and drain the shrimp in a colander. Transfer them to the ice bath to cool for 5 minutes, then drain them in the colander and set aside in the refrigerator. 5. Rinse out the inner pot and return it to the housing. Pour in 1 cup water and place the wire metal steam rack into the pot. Place the eggs on top of the steam rack. 6. Secure the lid and set the Pressure Release to Sealing. Press the Cancel button to reset the cooking program, then select the Egg, Pressure Cook, or Manual setting and set the cooking time for 5 minutes at high pressure. (The pot will take about 5 minutes to come up to pressure before the cooking program begins.) 7. While the eggs are cooking, prepare another ice bath. 8. When the cooking program ends, let the pressure release naturally for 5 minutes, then move the Pressure Release to Venting to release any remaining steam. Using tongs, transfer the eggs to the ice bath and let cool for 5 minutes.

To make the dressing:

1. In a small bowl, stir together the ketchup, mayonnaise, lemon juice, Worcestershire sauce, cayenne, ¼ teaspoon black pepper, and green onions. 2. Arrange the lettuce, cucumber, radishes, tomatoes, and avocado on individual plates or in large, shallow individual bowls. Mound the cooked shrimp in the center of each salad. Peel the eggs, quarter them lengthwise, and place the quarters around the shrimp. 3. Spoon the dressing over the salads and top with additional black pepper. Serve right away.

**Per Serving**

Calories: 407 | fat: 23g | protein: 35g | carbs: 16g | sugars: 10g | fiber: 6g | sodium: 1099mg

# Lemon-Pepper Salmon with Roasted Broccoli

### Prep time: 5 minutes | Cook time: 20 minutes | Serves 4

4 (6-ounce [170-g]) salmon fillets
Juice of 1 medium lemon (see Tips)
¼ teaspoon garlic salt or ¼ teaspoon sea salt
1 pound (454 g) broccoli florets
¼ teaspoon garlic powder

Cooking oil spray, as needed
½ teaspoon black pepper
mixed with ¼ teaspoon garlic powder
¼ teaspoon sea salt

1. Preheat the oven to 400°F (204°C). Line two large baking sheets with parchment paper. 2. Place the salmon on the first prepared baking sheet, making sure the fillets are evenly spaced. Spray the salmon with the cooking oil spray. Drizzle the lemon juice over each of the salmon fillets, then sprinkle the black pepper and garlic salt over each fillet. 3. Spread the broccoli out evenly on the second prepared baking sheet and spray the broccoli with cooking oil spray. Sprinkle the sea salt and garlic powder over the broccoli. 4. Place both baking sheets in the oven. Bake the salmon for 10 to 12 minutes, until it is light brown, depending on your preferred doneness and the thickness of the fillets. Bake the broccoli for 12 minutes, until the edges are slightly crispy. Serve the salmon and broccoli immediately.

**Per Serving**
Calorie: 353 | fat: 19g | protein: 37g | carbs: 9g | sugars: 2g | fiber: 3g | sodium: 406mg

# Asian Cod with Brown Rice, Asparagus, and Mushrooms

### Prep time: 5 minutes | Cook time: 25 minutes | Serves 2

¾ cup Minute brand brown rice
Two 5-ounce skinless cod fillets
1 tablespoon fresh lemon juice
1 tablespoon extra-virgin olive oil or
1 tablespoon unsalted butter, cut into 8 pieces
4 ounces shiitake mushrooms,
stems removed and sliced
Lemon wedges for serving

½ cup water
1 tablespoon soy sauce or tamari
½ teaspoon peeled and grated fresh ginger
2 green onions, white and green parts, thinly sliced
12 ounces asparagus, trimmed
⅛ teaspoon fine sea salt
⅛ teaspoon freshly ground black pepper

1. Pour 1 cup water into the Instant Pot. Have ready two-tier stackable stainless-steel containers. 2. In one of the containers, combine the rice and ½ cup water, then gently shake the container to spread the rice into an even layer, making sure all of the grains are submerged. Place the fish fillets on top of the rice. In a small bowl, stir together the soy sauce, lemon juice, and ginger. Pour the soy sauce mixture over the fillets. Drizzle 1 teaspoon olive oil on each fillet (or top with two pieces of the butter), and sprinkle the green onions on and around the fish. 3. In the second container, arrange the asparagus in the center in as even a layer as possible. Place the mushrooms on either side of the asparagus. Drizzle with the remaining 2 teaspoons olive oil (or put the remaining six pieces butter on top of the asparagus, spacing them evenly). Sprinkle the salt and pepper evenly over the vegetables. 4. Place the container with the rice and fish on the bottom and the vegetable container on top. Cover the top container with its lid and then latch the containers together. Grasping the handle, lower the containers into the Instant Pot. 5. Secure the lid and set the Pressure Release to Sealing. Select the Pressure Cook or Manual setting and set the cooking time for 15 minutes at high pressure. (The pot will take about 10 minutes to come up to pressure before the cooking program begins.) 6. When the cooking program ends, let the pressure release naturally for 5 minutes, then move the Pressure Release to Venting to release any remaining steam. Open the pot and, wearing heat-resistant mitts, lift out the stacked containers. Unlatch, unstack, and open the containers, taking care not to get burned by the steam. 7. Transfer the vegetables, rice, and fish to plates and serve right away, with the lemon wedges on the side.

**Per Serving**
Calories: 344 | fat: 11g | protein: 27g | carbs: 46g | sugars: 6g | fiber: 7g | sodium: 637mg

# Lemon Pepper Tilapia with Broccoli and Carrots

## Prep time: 0 minutes | Cook time: 15 minutes | Serves 4

| | |
|---|---|
| 1 pound tilapia fillets | 1 teaspoon lemon pepper seasoning |
| ¼ teaspoon fine sea salt | 2 tablespoons extra-virgin olive oil |
| 2 garlic cloves, minced | 1 small yellow onion, sliced |
| ½ cup low-sodium vegetable broth | 2 tablespoons fresh lemon juice |
| 1 pound broccoli crowns, cut into bite-size florets | 8 ounces carrots, cut into ¼-inch thick rounds |

1. Sprinkle the tilapia fillets all over with the lemon pepper seasoning and salt. 2. Select the Sauté setting on the Instant Pot and heat the oil and garlic for 2 minutes, until the garlic is bubbling but not browned. Add the onion and sauté for about 3 minutes more, until it begins to soften. 3. Pour in the broth and lemon juice, then use a wooden spoon to nudge any browned bits from the bottom of the pot. Using tongs, add the fish fillets to the pot in a single layer; it's fine if they overlap slightly. Place the broccoli and carrots on top. 4. Secure the lid and set the Pressure Release to Sealing. Press the Cancel button to reset the cooking program, then select the Pressure Cook or Manual setting and set the cooking time for 1 minute at low pressure. (The pot will take about 10 minutes to come up to pressure before the cooking program begins.) 5. When the cooking program ends, let the pressure release naturally for 10 minutes (don't open the pot before the 10 minutes are up, even if the float valve has gone down), then move the Pressure Release to Venting to release any remaining steam. Open the pot. Use a fish spatula to transfer the vegetables and fillets to plates. Serve right away.

**Per Serving**

Calories: 243 | fat: 9g | protein: 28g | carbs: 15g | sugars: 4g | fiber: 5g | sodium: 348mg

# Citrus-Glazed Salmon

## Prep time: 10 minutes | Cook time: 13 to 17 minutes | Serves 4

| | |
|---|---|
| 2 medium limes | 1 small orange |
| ⅓ cup agave syrup | 1 teaspoon salt |
| 1 teaspoon pepper | 4 cloves garlic, finely chopped |
| 1¼ pounds salmon fillet, cut into 4 pieces | 2 tablespoons sliced green onions |
| 1 lime slice, cut into 4 wedges | 1 orange slice, cut into 4 wedges |
| Hot cooked orzo pasta or rice, if desired | |

1. Heat oven to 400°F. Line 15x10x1-inch pan with cooking parchment paper or foil. In small bowl, grate lime peel from limes. Squeeze enough lime juice to equal 2 tablespoons; add to peel in bowl. Grate orange peel from oranges into bowl. Squeeze enough orange juice to equal 2 tablespoons; add to peel mixture. Stir in agave syrup, salt, pepper and garlic. In small cup, measure ¼ cup citrus mixture for salmon (reserve remaining citrus mixture). 2. Place salmon fillets in pan, skin side down. Using ¼ cup citrus mixture, brush tops and sides of salmon. Bake 13 to 17 minutes or until fish flakes easily with fork. Lift salmon pieces from skin with metal spatula onto serving plate. Sprinkle with green onions. Top each fish fillet with lime and orange wedges. Serve each fillet with 3 tablespoons reserved sauce and rice.

**Per Serving**

Calories: 320 | fat: 8g | protein: 31g | carbs: 30g | sugars: 23g | fiber: 3g | sodium: 680mg

# Tomato Tuna Melts

## Prep time: 5 minutes | Cook time: 5 minutes | Serves 2

1 (5-ounce) can chunk light tuna
packed in water, drained
2 tablespoons finely chopped celery
Pinch cayenne pepper
½ cup shredded cheddar cheese

2 tablespoons plain nonfat Greek yogurt
2 teaspoons freshly squeezed lemon juice
1 tablespoon finely chopped red onion
1 large tomato, cut into ¾-inch-thick rounds

1. Preheat the broiler to high. 2. In a medium bowl, combine the tuna, yogurt, lemon juice, celery, red onion, and cayenne pepper. Stir well. 3. Arrange the tomato slices on a baking sheet. Top each with some tuna salad and cheddar cheese. 4. Broil for 3 to 4 minutes until the cheese is melted and bubbly. Serve.
**Per Serving**
Calories: 243 | fat: 10g | protein: 30g | carbs: 7g | sugars: 2g | fiber: 1g | sodium: 444mg

# Ginger-Garlic Cod Cooked in Paper

## Prep time: 10 minutes | Cook time: 15 minutes | Serves 4

1 chard bunch, stemmed, leaves and stems
1 red bell pepper, seeded and cut into strips
1 tablespoon grated fresh ginger
2 tablespoons white wine vinegar
1 tablespoon honey

cut into thin strips
1 pound cod fillets cut into 4 pieces
3 garlic cloves, minced
2 tablespoons low-sodium tamari
or gluten-free soy sauce

1. Preheat the oven to 425°F. 2. Cut four pieces of parchment paper, each about 16 inches wide. Lay the four pieces out on a large workspace. 3. On each piece of paper, arrange a small pile of chard leaves and stems, topped by several strips of bell pepper. Top with a piece of cod. 4. In a small bowl, mix the ginger, garlic, vinegar, tamari, and honey. Top each piece of fish with one-fourth of the mixture. 5. Fold the parchment paper over so the edges overlap. Fold the edges over several times to secure the fish in the packets. Carefully place the packets on a large baking sheet. 6. Bake for 12 minutes. Carefully open the packets, allowing steam to escape, and serve.
**Per Serving**
Calories: 118 | fat: 1g | protein: 19g | carbs: 9g | sugars: 6g | fiber: 1g | sodium: 715mg

# Cobia with Lemon-Caper Sauce

## Prep time: 25 minutes | Cook time: 10 minutes | Serves 4

⅓ cup all-purpose flour
¼ teaspoon pepper
2 tablespoons olive oil
½ cup reduced-sodium chicken broth
1 tablespoon capers, rinsed, drained

¼ teaspoon salt
1¼ pounds cobia or sea bass fillets, cut into 4 pieces
⅓ cup dry white wine
2 tablespoons lemon juice
1 tablespoon chopped fresh parsley

1. In shallow dish, stir flour, salt and pepper. Coat cobia pieces in flour mixture (reserve remaining flour mixture). In 12-inch nonstick skillet, heat oil over medium-high heat. Place coated cobia in oil. Cook 8 to 10 minutes, turning halfway through cooking, until fish flakes easily with fork; remove from heat. Lift fish from skillet to serving platter with slotted spatula (do not discard drippings); keep warm. 2. Heat skillet (with drippings) over medium heat. Stir in 1 tablespoon reserved flour mixture; cook and stir 30 seconds. Stir in wine; cook about 30 seconds or until thickened and slightly reduced. Stir in chicken broth and lemon juice; cook and stir 1 to 2 minutes until sauce is smooth and slightly thickened. Stir in capers. 3. Serve sauce over cobia; sprinkle with parsley.
**Per Serving**
Calories: 230 | fat: 9g | protein: 28g | carbs: 9g | sugars: 0g | fiber: 0g | sodium: 400mg

# Scallops and Asparagus Skillet

## Prep time: 10 minutes | Cook time: 15 minutes | Serves 4

3 teaspoons extra-virgin olive oil, divided

1 tablespoon butter

1 pound sea scallops

Juice of 1 lemon

¼ teaspoon freshly ground black pepper

1 pound asparagus, trimmed and cut into 2-inch segments

¼ cup dry white wine

2 garlic cloves, minced

1. In a large skillet, heat 1½ teaspoons of oil over medium heat. 2. Add the asparagus and sauté for 5 to 6 minutes until just tender, stirring regularly. Remove from the skillet and cover with aluminum foil to keep warm. 3. Add the remaining 1½ teaspoons of oil and the butter to the skillet. When the butter is melted and sizzling, place the scallops in a single layer in the skillet. Cook for about 3 minutes on one side until nicely browned. Use tongs to gently loosen and flip the scallops, and cook on the other side for another 3 minutes until browned and cooked through. Remove and cover with foil to keep warm. 4. In the same skillet, combine the wine, lemon juice, garlic, and pepper. Bring to a simmer for 1 to 2 minutes, stirring to mix in any browned pieces left in the pan. 5. Return the asparagus and the cooked scallops to the skillet to coat with the sauce. Serve warm.

**Per Serving**

Calories: 252 | fat: 7g | protein: 26g | carbs: 15g | sugars: 3g | fiber: 2g | sodium: 493mg

# Calypso Shrimp with Black Bean Salsa

## Prep time: 25 minutes | Cook time: 5 minutes | Serves 4

**Shrimp**

½ teaspoon grated lime peel

1 tablespoon canola oil

1 clove garlic, finely chopped

1 tablespoon lime juice

1 teaspoon finely chopped gingerroot

1 pound uncooked deveined peeled large shrimp, thawed if frozen

**Salsa**

1 can (15 ounces) black beans, drained, rinsed

1 small red bell pepper, chopped (½ cup)

1 tablespoon chopped fresh cilantro

1 to 2 tablespoons lime juice

¼ teaspoon ground red pepper (cayenne)

1 medium mango, peeled, pitted and chopped (1 cup)

2 medium green onions, sliced (2 tablespoons)

½ teaspoon grated lime peel

1 tablespoon red wine vinegar

1. In medium glass or plastic bowl, mix lime peel, lime juice, oil, gingerroot and garlic. Stir in shrimp; let stand 15 minutes. 2. Meanwhile, in medium bowl, mix salsa ingredients. 3. In 10-inch skillet, cook shrimp over medium-high heat about 5 minutes, turning once, until pink. Serve with salsa.

**Per Serving**

Calories: 300| fat: 5g | protein: 26g | carbs: 37g | sugars: 7g | fiber: 12g | sodium: 190mg

# Roasted Halibut with Red Peppers, Green Beans, and Onions

## Prep time: 10 minutes | Cook time: 15 minutes | Serves 4

1 pound green beans, trimmed

1 onion, sliced

3 garlic cloves, minced

1 teaspoon dried dill

4 (4-ounce) halibut fillets

¼ teaspoon freshly ground black pepper

2 red bell peppers, seeded and cut into strips

Zest and juice of 2 lemons

2 tablespoons extra-virgin olive oil

1 teaspoon dried oregano

½ teaspoon salt

1. Preheat the oven to 400°F. Line a baking sheet with parchment paper. 2. In a large bowl, toss the green beans, bell peppers, onion, lemon zest and juice, garlic, olive oil, dill, and oregano. 3. Use a slotted spoon to transfer the vegetables to the prepared baking sheet in a single layer, leaving the juice behind in the bowl. 4. Gently place the halibut fillets in the bowl, and coat in the juice. Transfer the fillets to the baking sheet, nestled between the vegetables, and drizzle them with any juice left in the bowl. Sprinkle the vegetables and halibut with the salt and pepper. 5. Bake for 15 to 20 minutes until the vegetables are just tender and the fish flakes apart easily.

**Per Serving**

Calories: 234 | fat: 9g | protein: 24g | carbs: 16g | sugars: 8g | fiber: 5g | sodium: 349mg

# Roasted Salmon with Salsa Verde

## Prep time: 5 minutes | Cook time: 25 minutes | Serves 4

Nonstick cooking spray

½ onion, quartered

1 garlic clove, unpeeled

½ teaspoon salt, divided

¼ teaspoon freshly ground black pepper

Juice of 1 lime

8 ounces tomatillos, husks removed

1 jalapeño or serrano pepper, seeded

1 teaspoon extra-virgin olive oil

4 (4-ounce) wild-caught salmon fillets

¼ cup chopped fresh cilantro

1. Preheat the oven to 425°F. Spray a baking sheet with nonstick cooking spray. 2. In a large bowl, toss the tomatillos, onion, jalapeño, garlic, olive oil, and ¼ teaspoon of salt to coat. Arrange in a single layer on the prepared baking sheet, and roast for about 10 minutes until just softened. Transfer to a dish or plate and set aside. 3. Arrange the salmon fillets skin-side down on the same baking sheet, and season with the remaining ¼ teaspoon of salt and the pepper. Bake for 12 to 15 minutes until the fish is firm and flakes easily. 4. Meanwhile, peel the roasted garlic and place it and the roasted vegetables in a blender or food processor. Add a scant ¼ cup of water to the jar, and process until smooth. 5. Add the cilantro and lime juice and process until smooth. Serve the salmon topped with the salsa verde.

**Per Serving**

Calories: 199 | fat: 9g | protein: 23g | carbs: 6g | sugars: 3g | fiber: 2g | sodium: 295mg

# Halibut with Lime and Cilantro

## Prep time: 30 minutes | Cook time: 10 to 20 minutes | Serves 2

2 tablespoons lime juice
1 teaspoon olive or canola oil
2 halibut or salmon steaks (about ¾ pound)
½ cup chunky-style salsa

1 tablespoon chopped fresh cilantro
1 clove garlic, finely chopped
Freshly ground pepper to taste

1. In shallow glass or plastic dish or in resealable food-storage plastic bag, mix lime juice, cilantro, oil and garlic. Add halibut, turning several times to coat with marinade. Cover; refrigerate 15 minutes, turning once. 2. Heat gas or charcoal grill. Remove halibut from marinade; discard marinade. 3. Place halibut on grill over medium heat. Cover grill; cook 10 to 20 minutes, turning once, until halibut flakes easily with fork. Sprinkle with pepper. Serve with salsa.
**Per Serving**
Calories: 190 | fat: 4.5g | protein: 32g | carbs: 6g | sugars: 2g | fiber: 0g | sodium: 600mg

# Roasted Tilapia and Vegetables

## Prep time: 15 minutes | Cook time: 20 minutes | Serves 4

½ pound fresh asparagus spears, trimmed, halved
1 red bell pepper, cut into ½-inch strips
1 large onion, cut into ½-inch wedges
2 teaspoons Montreal steak seasoning
2 teaspoons butter or margarine, melted

2 small zucchini, halved lengthwise, cut into ½-inch pieces
1 tablespoon olive oil
4 tilapia fillets (about 1½ pounds)
½ teaspoon paprika

1. Heat oven to 450°F. In large bowl, toss asparagus, zucchini, bell pepper, onion and oil. Sprinkle with 1 teaspoon of the steak seasoning; toss to coat. Spread vegetables in ungreased 15x10x1-inch pan. Place on lower oven rack; roast 5 minutes. 2. Meanwhile, spray 13x9-inch (3-quart) glass baking dish with cooking spray. Pat tilapia fillets dry with paper towels. Brush with butter; sprinkle with remaining 1 teaspoon steak seasoning and the paprika. Place in baking dish. 3. Place baking dish on middle oven rack. Roast fish and vegetables 17 to 18 minutes longer or until fish flakes easily with fork and vegetables are tender.
**Per Serving**
Calories: 250 | fat: 8g | protein: 35g | carbs: 10g | sugars: 5g | fiber: 3g | sodium: 160mg

# Whole Veggie-Stuffed Trout

## Prep time: 10 minutes | Cook time: 25 minutes | Serves 2

Nonstick cooking spray
1 tablespoon extra-virgin olive oil
¼ teaspoon salt
½ red bell pepper, seeded and thinly sliced
2 or 3 shiitake mushrooms, sliced
1 lemon, sliced

2 (8-ounce) whole trout fillets, dressed (cleaned but with bones and skin intact)
⅛ teaspoon freshly ground black pepper
1 small onion, thinly sliced
1 poblano pepper, seeded and thinly sliced

1. Preheat the oven to 425°F. Spray a baking sheet with nonstick cooking spray. 2. Rub both trout, inside and out, with the olive oil, then season with the salt and pepper. 3. In a large bowl, combine the bell pepper, onion, mushrooms, and poblano pepper. Stuff half of this mixture into the cavity of each fish. Top the mixture with 2 or 3 lemon slices inside each fish. 4. Arrange the fish on the prepared baking sheet side by side and roast for 25 minutes until the fish is cooked through and the vegetables are tender.
**Per Serving**
Calories: 452 | fat: 22g | protein: 49g | carbs: 14g | sugars: 2g | fiber: 3g | sodium: 357mg

# Fish Tacos

**Prep time: 5 minutes | Cook time: 10 minutes | Serves 4**

**For the tacos**
2 tablespoons extra-virgin olive oil
8 (10-inch) yellow corn tortillas
¼ cup chopped fresh cilantro
4 (6-ounce) cod fillets
2 cups packaged shredded cabbage
4 lime wedges

**For the sauce**
½ cup plain low-fat Greek yogurt
½ teaspoon garlic powder
⅓ cup low-fat mayonnaise
½ teaspoon ground cumin

To make the tacos:

Heat a medium skillet over medium-low heat. When hot, pour the oil into the skillet, then add the fish and cover. Cook for 4 minutes, then flip and cook for 4 minutes more. 2. Top each tortilla with one-eighth of the cabbage, sauce, cilantro, and fish. Finish each taco with a squeeze of lime.

To make the sauce:

1. In a small bowl, whisk together the yogurt, mayonnaise, garlic powder, and cumin.

**Per Serving**
Calories: 373 | fat: 13g | protein: 36g | carbs: 30g | sugars: 4g | fiber: 4g | sodium: 342mg

# Grilled Fish with Jicama Salsa

**Prep time: 15 minutes | Cook time: 10 minutes | Serves 6**

**Jicama Salsa**
2 cups chopped peeled jicama (¾ pound)
1 medium orange, peeled, chopped (¾ cup)
½ teaspoon chili powder
1 tablespoon lime juice
1 medium cucumber, peeled, chopped (1 cup)
1 tablespoon chopped fresh cilantro or parsley
¼ teaspoon salt

**Fish**
1½ pounds swordfish, tuna or marlin steaks,
¾ to 1 inch thick
¼ teaspoon salt
2 tablespoons olive or canola oil
1 tablespoon lime juice
⅛ teaspoon crushed red pepper

1. In medium bowl, mix salsa ingredients. Cover and refrigerate at least 2 hours to blend flavors. 2. If fish steaks are large, cut into 6 serving pieces. Mix oil, lime juice, salt and red pepper in shallow glass or plastic dish or heavy-duty resealable food-storage plastic bag. Add fish; turn to coat with marinade. Cover dish or seal bag; refrigerate 30 minutes. 3. Heat charcoal or gas grill for direct heat. Remove fish from marinade; reserve marinade. Cover and grill fish 5 to 6 inches from medium heat about 10 minutes, brushing 2 or 3 times with marinade and turning once, until fish flakes easily with fork. Discard any remaining marinade. Serve fish with salsa.

**Per Serving**
Calories: 200 | fat: 10g | protein: 20g | carbs: 7g | sugars: 2g | fiber: 3g | sodium: 250mg

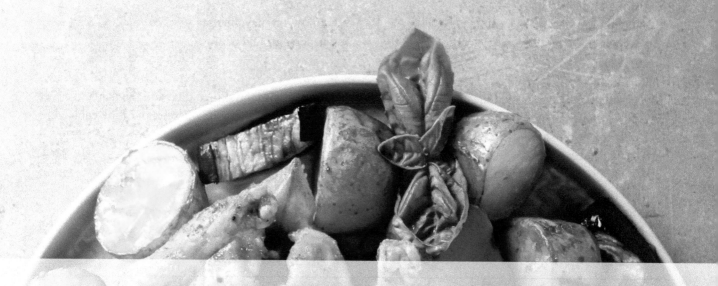
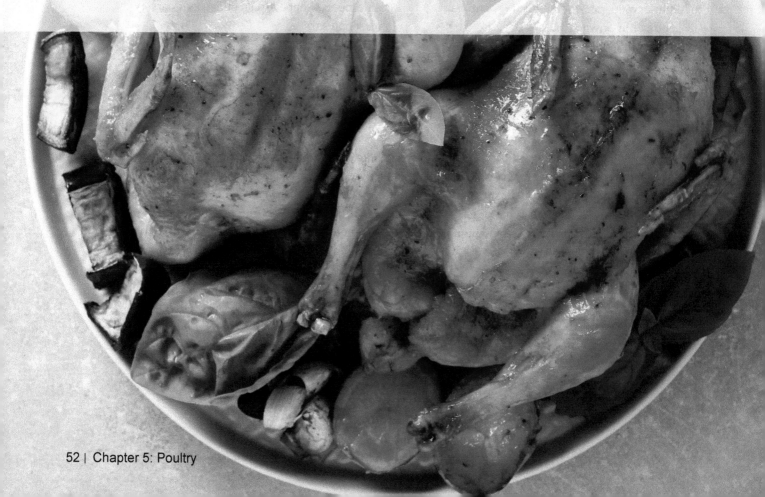

# Chapter 5   Poultry

# Unstuffed Peppers with Ground Turkey and Quinoa

## Prep time: 0 minutes | Cook time: 35 minutes | Serves 8

2 tablespoons extra-virgin olive oil

2 celery stalks, diced

2 pounds 93 percent lean ground turkey

½ teaspoon freshly ground black pepper

¼ teaspoon cayenne pepper

1 cup low-sodium chicken broth

3 red, orange, and/or yellow bell peppers, seeded and cut into 1-inch squares

1½ tablespoons chopped fresh flat-leaf parsley

1 yellow onion, diced

2 garlic cloves, chopped

2 teaspoons Cajun seasoning blend (plus 1 teaspoon fine sea salt if using a salt-free blend)

1 cup quinoa, rinsed

One 14½-ounce can fire-roasted diced tomatoes and their liquid

1 green onion, white and green parts, thinly sliced

Hot sauce (such as Crystal or Frank's RedHot) for serving

1. Select the Sauté setting on the Instant Pot and heat the oil for 2 minutes. Add the onion, celery, and garlic and sauté for about 4 minutes, until the onion begins to soften. Add the turkey, Cajun seasoning, black pepper, and cayenne and sauté, using a wooden spoon or spatula to break up the meat as it cooks, for about 6 minutes, until cooked through and no streaks of pink remain. 2. Sprinkle the quinoa over the turkey in an even layer. Pour the broth and the diced tomatoes and their liquid over the quinoa, spreading the tomatoes on top. Sprinkle the bell peppers over the top in an even layer. 3. Secure the lid and set the Pressure Release to Sealing. Press the Cancel button to reset the cooking program, then select the Pressure Cook or Manual setting and set the cooking time for 8 minutes at high pressure. (The pot will take about 15 minutes to come up to pressure before the cooking program begins.) 4. When the cooking program ends, let the pressure release naturally for at least 15 minutes, then move the Pressure Release to Venting to release any remaining steam. Open the pot and sprinkle the green onion and parsley over the top in an even layer. 5. Spoon the unstuffed peppers into bowls, making sure to dig down to the bottom of the pot so each person gets an equal amount of peppers, quinoa, and meat. Serve hot, with hot sauce on the side.

**Per Serving**

Calories: 320 | fat: 14g | protein: 27g | carbs: 23g | sugars: 3g | fiber: 3g | sodium: 739mg

# Lemony Chicken Thighs

## Prep time: 15 minutes | Cook time: 15 minutes | Serves 3 to 5

1 cup low-sodium chicken bone broth

1 small onion, diced

Juice of 1 lemon

½ teaspoon salt

1 teaspoon True Lemon Lemon Pepper seasoning

¼ teaspoon oregano

5 frozen bone-in chicken thighs

5–6 cloves garlic, diced

2 tablespoons margarine, melted

¼ teaspoon black pepper

1 teaspoon parsley flakes

Rind of 1 lemon

1. Add the chicken bone broth into the inner pot of the Instant Pot. 2. Add the chicken thighs. 3. Add the onion and garlic. 4. Pour the fresh lemon juice in with the melted margarine. 5. Add the seasonings. 6. Lock the lid, make sure the vent is at sealing, then press the Poultry button. Set to 15 minutes. 7. When cook time is up, let the pressure naturally release for 3–5 minutes, then manually release the rest. 8. You can place these under the broiler for 2–3 minutes to brown. 9. Plate up and pour some of the sauce over top with fresh grated lemon rind.

**Per Serving**

Calories: 329 | fat: 24g | protein: 26g | carbs: 3g | sugars: 1g | fiber: 0g | sodium: 407mg

# Ann's Chicken Cacciatore

## Prep time: 25 minutes | Cook time: 3 to 9 minutes | Serves 8

1 large onion, thinly sliced
2 (6-ounce) cans tomato paste
1 teaspoon salt
¼ teaspoons pepper
1–2 teaspoons dried oregano
½ teaspoon celery seed, optional

3 pound chicken, cut up, skin removed, trimmed of fat
4-ounce can sliced mushrooms, drained
¼ cup dry white wine
1–2 garlic cloves, minced
½ teaspoon dried basil
1 bay leaf

1. In the inner pot of the Instant Pot, place the onion and chicken. 2. Combine remaining ingredients and pour over the chicken. 3. Secure the lid and make sure vent is at sealing. Cook on Slow Cook mode, low 7–9 hours, or high 3–4 hours.

**Per Serving**
Calories: 161 | fat: 4g | protein: 19g | carbs: 12g | sugars: 3g | fiber: 3g | sodium: 405mg

# Chicken in Mushroom Gravy

## Prep time: 10 minutes | Cook time: 10 minutes | Serves 6

6 (5 ounces each) boneless, skinless chicken-breast halves
10¾-ounce can 98% fat-free, reduced-sodium cream of mushroom soup

Salt and pepper to taste
¼ cup dry white wine or low-sodium chicken broth
4 ounces sliced mushrooms

1. Place chicken in the inner pot of the Instant Pot. Season with salt and pepper. 2. Combine wine and soup in a bowl, then pour over the chicken. Top with the mushrooms. 3. Secure the lid and make sure the vent is set to sealing. Set on Manual mode for 10 minutes. 4. When cooking time is up, let the pressure release naturally.

**Per Serving**
Calories: 204 | fat: 4g | protein: 34g | carbs: 6g | sugars: 1g | fiber: 1g | sodium: 320mg

# Turkey and Quinoa Caprese Casserole

## Prep time: 10 minutes | Cook time: 35 minutes | Serves 8

⅔ cup quinoa
Nonstick cooking spray
1 pound lean ground turkey
½ teaspoon salt
4 cups spinach leaves, finely sliced
¼ cup sliced fresh basil
2 large ripe tomatoes, sliced

1⅓ cups water
2 teaspoons extra-virgin olive oil
¼ cup chopped red onion
1 (15-ounce can) fire-roasted tomatoes, drained
3 garlic cloves, minced
¼ cup chicken or vegetable broth
4 ounces mozzarella cheese, thinly sliced

1. In a small pot, combine the quinoa and water. Bring to a boil, reduce the heat, cover, and simmer for 10 minutes. Turn off the heat, and let the quinoa sit for 5 minutes to absorb any remaining water. 2. Preheat the oven to 400°F. Spray a baking dish with nonstick cooking spray. 3. In a large skillet, heat the oil over medium heat. Add the turkey, onion, and salt. Cook until the turkey is cooked through and crumbled. 4. Add the tomatoes, spinach, garlic, and basil. Stir in the broth and cooked quinoa. Transfer the mixture to the prepared baking dish. Arrange the tomato and cheese slices on top. 5. Bake for 15 minutes until the cheese is melted and the tomatoes are softened. Serve.

**Per Serving**
Calories: 218 | fat: 9g | protein: 18g | carbs: 17g | sugars: 3g | fiber: 3g | sodium: 340mg

# Turkey Divan Casserole

## Prep time: 10 minutes | Cook time: 50 minutes | Serves 6

Nonstick cooking spray
1 pound turkey cutlets
¼ teaspoon freshly ground black pepper, divided
2 garlic cloves, minced
1 cup unsweetened plain almond milk
½ cup shredded Swiss cheese, divided
4 cups chopped broccoli

3 teaspoons extra-virgin olive oil, divided
Pinch salt
¼ cup chopped onion
2 tablespoons whole-wheat flour
1 cup low-sodium chicken broth
½ teaspoon dried thyme
¼ cup coarsely ground almonds

1. Preheat the oven to 375°F. Spray a baking dish with nonstick cooking spray. 2. In a skillet, heat 1 teaspoon of oil over medium heat. Season the turkey with the salt and ⅛ teaspoon of pepper. Sauté the turkey cutlets for 5 to 7 minutes on each side until cooked through. Transfer to a cutting board, cool briefly, and cut into bite-size pieces. 3. In the same pan, heat the remaining 2 teaspoons of oil over medium-high heat. Sauté the onion for 3 minutes until it begins to soften. Add the garlic and continue cooking for another minute. 4. Stir in the flour and mix well. Whisk in the almond milk, broth, and remaining ⅛ teaspoon of pepper, and continue whisking until smooth. Add ¼ cup of cheese and the thyme, and continue stirring until the cheese is melted. 5. In the prepared baking dish, arrange the broccoli on the bottom. Cover with half the sauce. Place the turkey pieces on top of the broccoli, and cover with the remaining sauce. Sprinkle with the remaining ¼ cup of cheese and the ground almonds. 6. Bake for 35 minutes until the sauce is bubbly and the top is browned.

**Per Serving**
Calories: 207 | fat: 8g | protein: 25g | carbs: 9g | sugars: 2g | fiber: 3g | sodium: 128mg

# Peanut Chicken Satay

## Prep time: 20 minutes | Cook time: 10 minutes | Serves 8

**For the peanut sauce:**
1 cup natural peanut butter
1 teaspoon red chili paste
Juice of 2 limes
**For the chicken:**
2 pounds boneless, skinless chicken thighs, trimmed of fat and cut into 1-inch pieces
1 teaspoon minced fresh ginger
1½ teaspoons ground coriander
½ teaspoon salt
Lettuce leaves, for serving

2 tablespoons low-sodium tamari or gluten-free soy sauce
1 tablespoon honey
½ cup hot water

½ cup plain nonfat Greek yogurt
2 garlic cloves, minced
½ onion, coarsely chopped
2 teaspoons ground cumin
1 teaspoon extra-virgin olive oil

**Make the peanut sauce:**
In a medium mixing bowl, combine the peanut butter, tamari, chili paste, honey, lime juice, and hot water. Mix until smooth. Set aside.

**Make the chicken:**
1. In a large mixing bowl, combine the chicken, yogurt, garlic, ginger, onion, coriander, cumin, and salt, and mix well. 2. Cover and marinate in the refrigerator for at least 2 hours. 3. Thread the chicken pieces onto bamboo skewers. 4. In a grill pan or large skillet, heat the oil. Cook the skewers for 3 to 5 minutes on each side until the pieces are cooked through. 5. Remove the chicken from the skewers and place a few pieces on each lettuce leaf. Drizzle with the peanut sauce and serve.

**Per Serving**
Calories: 386| fat: 26g | protein: 16g | carbs: 14g | sugars: 6g | fiber: 2g | sodium: 442mg

# Wild Rice and Turkey Casserole

## Prep time: 10 minutes | Cook time: 55 minutes | Serves 6

2 cups cut-up cooked turkey or chicken
⅓ cup fat-free (skim) milk
1 can (10.75 ounces) condensed 98% fat-free cream of mushroom soup
Additional green onions, if desired

2¼ cups boiling water
4 medium green onions, sliced (¼ cup)
1 package (6 ounces) original long-grain and wild rice mix

1. Heat oven to 350°F. In ungreased 2-quart casserole, mix all ingredients, including seasoning packet from rice mix. 2. Cover; bake 45 to 50 minutes or until rice is tender. Uncover; bake 10 to 15 minutes longer or until liquid is absorbed. Sprinkle with additional green onions.

**Per Serving**
Calories: 220 | fat: 4.5g | protein: 17g | carbs: 27g | sugars: 2g | fiber: 1g | sodium: 740mg

# Saffron-Spiced Chicken Breasts

## Prep time: 10 minutes | Cook time: 10 minutes | Serves 4

Pinch saffron (3 or 4 threads)
2 tablespoons water
3 garlic cloves, minced
Juice of ½ lemon
1 pound boneless, skinless chicken breasts, cut into 2-inch strips

½ cup plain nonfat yogurt
½ onion, chopped
2 tablespoons chopped fresh cilantro
½ teaspoon salt
1 tablespoon extra-virgin olive oil

1. In a blender jar, combine the saffron, yogurt, water, onion, garlic, cilantro, lemon juice, and salt. Pulse to blend. 2. In a large mixing bowl, combine the chicken and the yogurt sauce, and stir to coat. Cover and refrigerate for at least 1 hour or up to overnight. 3. In a large skillet, heat the oil over medium heat. Add the chicken pieces, shaking off any excess marinade. Discard the marinade. Cook the chicken pieces on each side for 5 minutes, flipping once, until cooked through and golden brown.

**Per Serving**
Calories: 155 | fat: 5g | protein: 26g | carbs: 3g | sugars: 1g | fiber: 0g | sodium: 501mg

# Baked Chicken Dijon

## Prep time: 25 minutes | Cook time: 40 minutes | Serves 6

3 cups uncooked bow-tie (farfalle) pasta (6 ounces)
2 cups cubed cooked chicken
1 can (10.75 ounces) condensed cream of chicken or cream of mushroom soup
1 tablespoon finely chopped onion

2 cups frozen broccoli cuts (from 12-ounce bag)
⅓ cup diced roasted red bell peppers (from 7-ounce jar)
⅓ cup reduced-sodium chicken broth (from 32-ounce carton)
3 tablespoons Dijon mustard
½ cup shredded Parmesan cheese

1. Heat oven to 375°F. Spray 2½-quart casserole with cooking spray. 2. Cook pasta as directed on package, adding broccoli for the last 2 minutes of cooking time; drain. In casserole, mix chicken and roasted peppers. In small bowl, mix soup, broth, mustard and onion; stir into chicken mixture. Stir in pasta and broccoli. Sprinkle with cheese. 3. Cover; bake about 30 minutes or until hot in center and cheese is melted.

**Per Serving**
Calories: 290 | fat: 9g | protein: 24g | carbs: 29g | sugars: 2g | fiber: 3g | sodium: 770mg

# Orange Chicken Thighs with Bell Peppers

## Prep time: 15 to 20 minutes | Cook time: 7 minutes | Serves 4 to 6

6 boneless skinless chicken thighs, cut into bite-sized pieces

½ teaspoon coconut aminos

Olive oil or cooking spray

1 onion, chopped

1 tablespoon green onion, chopped fine

½ teaspoon pink salt

1 teaspoon garlic powder

¼–½ teaspoon red pepper flakes

½ cup chicken bone broth or water

½ cup Seville orange spread (I use Crofter's brand)

2 packets crystallized True Orange flavoring

½ teaspoon True Orange Orange Ginger seasoning

¼ teaspoon Worcestershire sauce

2 cups bell pepper strips, any color combination (I used red)

3 cloves garlic, minced or chopped

½ teaspoon black pepper

1 teaspoon ground ginger

2 tablespoons tomato paste

1 tablespoon brown sugar substitute (I use Sukrin Gold)

1. Combine the chicken with the 2 packets of crystallized orange flavor, the orange ginger seasoning, the coconut aminos, and the Worcestershire sauce. Set aside. 2. Turn the Instant Pot to Sauté and add a touch of olive oil or cooking spray to the inner pot. Add in the orange ginger marinated chicken thighs. 3. Sauté until lightly browned. Add in the peppers, onion, green onion, garlic, and seasonings. Mix well. 4. Add the remaining ingredients; mix to combine. 5. Lock the lid, set the vent to sealing, set to 7 minutes. 6. Let the pressure release naturally for 2 minutes, then manually release the rest when cook time is up.

**Per Serving**

Calories: 120| fat: 2g | protein: 12g | carbs: 8g | sugars: 10g | fiber: 1.6g | sodium: 315mg

# Chicken Casablanca

## Prep time: 20 minutes | Cook time: 12 minutes | Serves 8

2 large onions, sliced

3 garlic cloves, minced

3 pounds skinless chicken pieces

2 large potatoes, unpeeled, diced

½ teaspoon salt

¼ teaspoon cinnamon

14½-ounce can chopped tomatoes

15-ounce can garbanzo beans, drained

1 teaspoon ground ginger

2 tablespoons canola oil, divided

3 large carrots, diced

½ teaspoon ground cumin

½ teaspoon pepper

2 tablespoons raisins

3 small zucchini, sliced

2 tablespoons chopped parsley

1. Using the Sauté function of the Instant Pot, cook the onions, ginger, and garlic in 1 tablespoon of the oil for 5 minutes, stirring constantly. Remove onions, ginger, and garlic from pot and set aside. 2. Brown the chicken pieces with the remaining oil, then add the cooked onions, ginger and garlic back in as well as all of the remaining ingredients, except the parsley. 3. Secure the lid and make sure vent is in the sealing position. Cook on Manual mode for 12 minutes. 4. When cook time is up, let the pressure release naturally for 5 minutes and then release the rest of the pressure manually.

**Per Serving**

Calories: 395 | fat: 10g | protein: 36g | carbs: 40g | sugars: 10g | fiber: 8g | sodium: 390mg

# Speedy Chicken Cacciatore

## Prep time: 5 minutes | Cook time: 30 minutes | Serves 6

2 pounds boneless, skinless chicken thighs
½ teaspoon freshly ground black pepper
3 garlic cloves, chopped
2 large yellow onions, sliced
½ cup dry red wine
½ teaspoon red pepper flakes (optional)
2 tablespoons tomato paste

1½ teaspoons fine sea salt
2 tablespoons extra-virgin olive oil
2 large red bell peppers, seeded and cut into
¼ by 2-inch strips
1½ teaspoons Italian seasoning
One 14½-ounce can diced tomatoes and their liquid
Cooked brown rice or whole-grain pasta for serving

1. Season the chicken thighs on both sides with 1 teaspoon of the salt and the black pepper. 2. Select the Sauté setting on the Instant Pot and heat the oil and garlic for 2 minutes, until the garlic is bubbling but not browned. Add the bell peppers, onions, and remaining ½ teaspoon salt and sauté for 3 minutes, until the onions begin to soften. Stir in the wine, Italian seasoning, and pepper flakes (if using). Using tongs, add the chicken to the pot, turning each piece to coat it in the wine and spices and nestling them in a single layer in the liquid. Pour the tomatoes and their liquid on top of the chicken and dollop the tomato paste on top. Do not stir them in. 3. Secure the lid and set the Pressure Release to Sealing. Press the Cancel button to reset the cooking program, then select the Poultry, Pressure Cook, or Manual setting and set the cooking time for 12 minutes at high pressure. (The pot will take about 15 minutes to come up to pressure before the cooking program begins.) 4. When the cooking program ends, perform a quick pressure release by moving the Pressure Release to Venting, or let the pressure release naturally. Open the pot and, using tongs, transfer the chicken and vegetables to a serving dish. 5. Spoon some of the sauce over the chicken and serve hot, with the rice on the side.

**Per Serving**
Calories: 297 | fat: 11g | protein: 32g | carbs: 16g | sugars: 3g | fiber: 3g | sodium: 772mg

# Grain-Free Parmesan Chicken

## Prep time: 5 minutes | Cook time: 20 minutes | Serves 4

1½ cups almond flour
1 tablespoon Italian seasoning
½ teaspoon black pepper
4 (6-ounce [170-g], ½-inch [13-mm]-thick) boneless,
skinless chicken breasts
2 tablespoons minced fresh herbs of choice (optional)

½ cup grated Parmesan cheese
1 teaspoon garlic powder
2 large eggs
½ cup no-added-sugar marinara sauce
½ cup shredded mozzarella cheese

1. Preheat the oven to 375°F (191°C). Line a large, rimmed baking sheet with parchment paper. 2. In a shallow dish, mix together the almond flour, Parmesan cheese, Italian seasoning, garlic powder, and black pepper. In another shallow dish, whisk the eggs. Dip a chicken breast into the egg wash, then gently shake off any extra egg. Dip the chicken breast into the almond flour mixture, coating it well. Place the chicken breast on the prepared baking sheet. Repeat this process with the remaining chicken breasts. 3. Bake the chicken for 15 to 20 minutes, or until the meat is no longer pink in the center. 4. Remove the chicken from the oven and flip each breast. Top each breast with 2 tablespoons of marinara sauce and 2 tablespoons of mozzarella cheese. 5. Increase the oven temperature to broil and place the chicken back in the oven. Broil it until the cheese is melted and just starting to brown. Carefully remove the chicken from the oven, top it with the herbs (if using), and let it rest for about 10 minutes before serving.

**Per Serving**
Calorie: 572 | fat: 32g | protein: 60g | carbs: 13g | sugars: 4g | fiber:5g | sodium: 560mg

# Sesame-Ginger Chicken Soba

## Prep time: 10 minutes | Cook time: 15 minutes | Serves 6

8 ounces soba noodles

¼ cup tahini

1 tablespoon reduced-sodium gluten-free soy sauce or tamari

⅓ cup water

1 scallions bunch, green parts only, cut into 1-inch segments

2 boneless, skinless chicken breasts, halved lengthwise

2 tablespoons rice vinegar

1 teaspoon toasted sesame oil

1 (1-inch) piece fresh ginger, finely grated

1 large cucumber, seeded and diced

1 tablespoon sesame seeds

1. Preheat the broiler to high. 2. Bring a large pot of water to a boil. Add the noodles and cook until tender, according to the package directions. Drain and rinse the noodles in cool water. 3. On a baking sheet, arrange the chicken in a single layer. Broil for 5 to 7 minutes on each side, depending on the thickness, until the chicken is cooked through and its juices run clear. Use two forks to shred the chicken. 4. In a small bowl, combine the tahini, rice vinegar, soy sauce, sesame oil, ginger, and water. Whisk to combine. 5. In a large bowl, toss the shredded chicken, noodles, cucumber, and scallions. Pour the tahini sauce over the noodles and toss to combine. Served sprinkled with the sesame seeds.

**Per Serving**

Calories: 251 | fat: 8g | protein: 16g | carbs: 35g | sugars: 2g | fiber: 2g | sodium: 482mg

# Teriyaki Turkey Meatballs

## Prep time: 20 minutes | Cook time: 20 minutes | Serves 6

1 pound lean ground turkey

1 egg

2 garlic cloves, minced

2 tablespoons reduced-sodium tamari or gluten-free soy sauce

1 teaspoon toasted sesame oil

¼ cup finely chopped scallions, both white and green parts

1 teaspoon grated fresh ginger

1 tablespoon honey

2 teaspoons mirin

1. Preheat the oven to 400°F. Line a baking sheet with parchment paper. 2. In a large mixing bowl, combine the turkey, scallions, egg, garlic, ginger, tamari, honey, mirin, and sesame oil. Mix well. 3. Using your hands, form the meat mixture into balls about the size of a tablespoon. Arrange on the prepared baking sheet. 4. Bake for 10 minutes, flip with a spatula, and continue baking for an additional 10 minutes until the meatballs are cooked through.

**Per Serving**

Calories: 153 | fat: 8g | protein: 16g | carbs: 5g | sugars: 4g | fiber: 0g | sodium: 270mg

# Pulled BBQ Chicken and Texas-Style Cabbage Slaw

## Prep time: 5 minutes | Cook time: 20 minutes | Serves 6

Chicken
¼ teaspoon fine sea salt
2 bay leaves
Cabbage Slaw
½ head red or green cabbage, thinly sliced
2 jalapeño chiles, seeded and cut into narrow strips
1 large Fuji or Gala apple, julienned
3 tablespoons fresh lime juice
½ teaspoon ground cumin
¾ cup low-sugar or unsweetened barbecue sauce

1 cup water
3 garlic cloves, peeled
2 pounds boneless, skinless chicken thighs
(see Note)
1 red bell pepper, seeded and thinly sliced
2 carrots, julienned
½ cup chopped fresh cilantro
3 tablespoons extra-virgin olive oil
¼ teaspoon fine sea salt
Cornbread, for serving

**To make the chicken:**

Combine the water, salt, garlic, bay leaves, and chicken thighs in the Instant Pot, arranging the chicken in a single layer. 2. Secure the lid and set the Pressure Release to Sealing. Select the Poultry, Pressure Cook, or Manual setting and set the cooking time for 10 minutes at high pressure. (The pot will take about 10 minutes to come up to pressure before the cooking program begins.)

**To make the slaw:**

1. While the chicken is cooking, in a large bowl, combine the cabbage, bell pepper, jalapeños, carrots, apple, cilantro, lime juice, oil, cumin, and salt and toss together until the vegetables and apples are evenly coated. 2. When the cooking program ends, perform a quick pressure release by moving the Pressure Release to Venting, or let the pressure release naturally. Open the pot and, using tongs, transfer the chicken to a cutting board. Using two forks, shred the chicken into bite-size pieces. Wearing heat-resistant mitts, lift out the inner pot and discard the cooking liquid. Return the inner pot to the housing. 3. Return the chicken to the pot and stir in the barbecue sauce. You can serve it right away or heat it for a minute or two on the Sauté setting, then return the pot to its Keep Warm setting until ready to serve. 6. Divide the chicken and slaw evenly among six plates. Serve with wedges of cornbread on the side.

**Per Serving**

Calories: 320 | fat: 14g | protein: 32g | carbs: 18g | sugars: 7g | fiber: 4g | sodium: 386mg

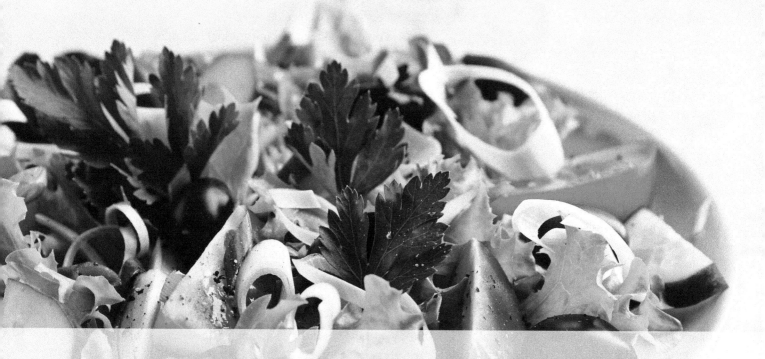

# Chapter 6 Salads

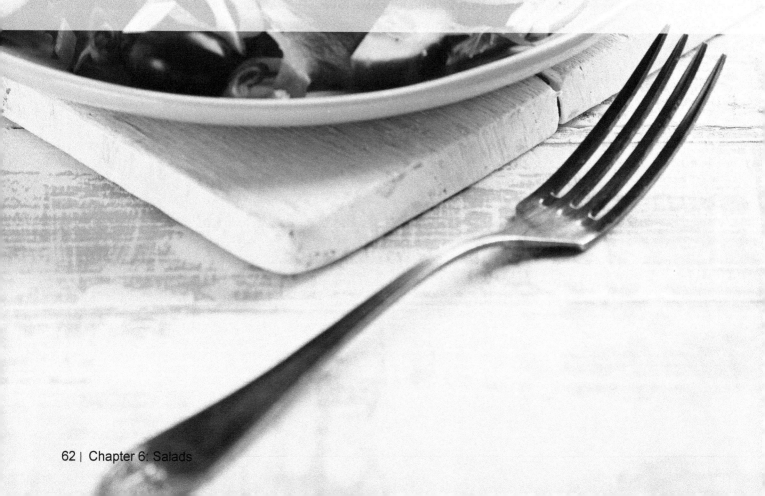

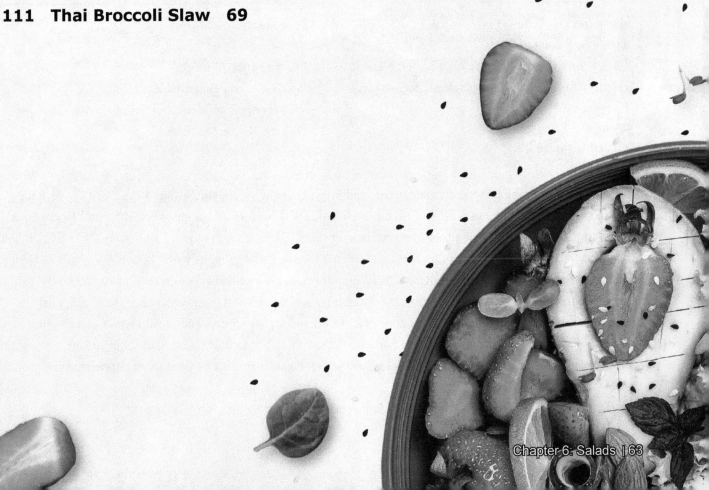

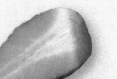

# Warm Barley and Squash Salad with Balsamic Vinaigrette

## Prep time: 20 minutes | Cook time: 40 minutes | Serves 8

| | |
|---|---|
| 1 small butternut squash | 3 teaspoons plus 2 tablespoons extra-virgin olive oil, divided |
| 2 cups broccoli florets | |
| 1 cup pearl barley | 1 cup toasted chopped walnuts |
| 2 cups baby kale | ½ red onion, sliced |
| 2 tablespoons balsamic vinegar | 2 garlic cloves, minced |
| ½ teaspoon salt | ¼ teaspoon freshly ground black pepper |

1. Preheat the oven to 400°F. Line a baking sheet with parchment paper. 2. Peel and seed the squash, and cut it into dice. In a large bowl, toss the squash with 2 teaspoons of olive oil. Transfer to the prepared baking sheet and roast for 20 minutes. 3. While the squash is roasting, toss the broccoli in the same bowl with 1 teaspoon of olive oil. After 20 minutes, flip the squash and push it to one side of the baking sheet. Add the broccoli to the other side and continue to roast for 20 more minutes until tender. 4. While the veggies are roasting, in a medium pot, cover the barley with several inches of water. Bring to a boil, then reduce the heat, cover, and simmer for 30 minutes until tender. Drain and rinse. 5. Transfer the barley to a large bowl, and toss with the cooked squash and broccoli, walnuts, kale, and onion. 6. In a small bowl, mix the remaining 2 tablespoons of olive oil, balsamic vinegar, garlic, salt, and pepper. Toss the salad with the dressing and serve.

**Per Serving**

Calories: 274 | fat: 15g | protein: 6g | carbs: 32g | sugars: 3g | fiber: 7g | sodium: 144mg

# Salmon, Quinoa, and Avocado Salad

## Prep time: 15 minutes | Cook time: 20 minutes | Serves 4

| | |
|---|---|
| ½ cup quinoa | 1 cup water |
| 4 (4-ounce) salmon fillets | 1 pound asparagus, trimmed |
| 1 teaspoon extra-virgin olive oil, plus 2 tablespoons | ½ teaspoon salt, divided |
| ½ teaspoon freshly ground black pepper, divided | ¼ teaspoon red pepper flakes |
| 1 avocado, chopped | ¼ cup chopped scallions, both white and green parts |
| ¼ cup chopped fresh cilantro | 1 tablespoon minced fresh oregano |
| Juice of 1 lime | |

1. In a small pot, combine the quinoa and water, and bring to a boil over medium-high heat. Cover, reduce the heat, and simmer for 15 minutes. 2. Preheat the oven to 425°F. Line a large baking sheet with parchment paper. 3. Arrange the salmon on one side of the prepared baking sheet. Toss the asparagus with 1 teaspoon of olive oil, and arrange on the other side of the baking sheet. Season the salmon and asparagus with ¼ teaspoon of salt, ¼ teaspoon of pepper, and the red pepper flakes. Roast for 12 minutes until browned and cooked through. 4. While the fish and asparagus are cooking, in a large mixing bowl, gently toss the cooked quinoa, avocado, scallions, cilantro, and oregano. Add the remaining 2 tablespoons of olive oil and the lime juice, and season with the remaining ¼ teaspoon of salt and ¼ teaspoon of pepper. 5. Break the salmon into pieces, removing the skin and any bones, and chop the asparagus into bite-sized pieces. Fold into the quinoa and serve warm or at room temperature.

**Per Serving**

Calorie: 397 | fat: 22g | protein: 29g | carbs: 23g | sugars: 3g | fiber: 8g | sodium: 292mg

# Roasted Asparagus–Berry Salad

## Prep time: 10 minutes | Cook time: 18 minutes | Serves 4

1 pound fresh asparagus spears
2 tablespoons chopped pecans
4 cups mixed salad greens
Cracked pepper, if desired

Cooking spray
1 cup sliced fresh strawberries
¼ cup fat-free balsamic vinaigrette dressing

1. Heat oven to 400°F. Line 15x10x1-inch pan with foil; spray with cooking spray. Break off tough ends of asparagus as far down as stalks snap easily. Cut into 1-inch pieces. 2. Place asparagus in single layer in pan; spray with cooking spray. Place pecans in another shallow pan. 3. Bake pecans 5 to 6 minutes or until golden brown, stirring occasionally. Bake asparagus 10 to 12 minutes or until crisp-tender. Cool pecans and asparagus 8 to 10 minutes or until room temperature. 4. In medium bowl, mix asparagus, pecans, strawberries, greens and dressing. Sprinkle with pepper.

**Per Serving**

Calorie: 90 | fat: 3g | protein: 4g | carbs: 11g | sugars: 6g | fiber: 4g | sodium: 180mg

# Blueberry and Chicken Salad on a Bed of Greens

## Prep time: 10 minutes | Cook time: 0 minutes | Serves 4

2 cups chopped cooked chicken
¼ cup finely chopped almonds
¼ cup finely chopped red onion
1 tablespoon chopped fresh cilantro
¼ teaspoon salt
8 cups salad greens (baby spinach, spicy greens, romaine)

1 cup fresh blueberries
1 celery stalk, finely chopped
1 tablespoon chopped fresh basil
½ cup plain, nonfat Greek yogurt or vegan mayonnaise
¼ teaspoon freshly ground black pepper

1. In a large mixing bowl, combine the chicken, blueberries, almonds, celery, onion, basil, and cilantro. Toss gently to mix. 2. In a small bowl, combine the yogurt, salt, and pepper. Add to the chicken salad and stir to combine. 3. Arrange 2 cups of salad greens on each of 4 plates and divide the chicken salad among the plates to serve.

**Per Serving**

Calories: 207 | fat: 6g | protein: 28g | carbs: 11g | sugars: 6g | fiber: 3g | sodium: 235mg

# Cabbage Slaw Salad

## Prep time: 15 minutes | Cook time: 0 minutes | Serves 6

2 cups finely chopped green cabbage
2 cups grated carrots
2 tablespoons extra-virgin olive oil
1 teaspoon honey
¼ teaspoon salt

2 cups finely chopped red cabbage
3 scallions, both white and green parts, sliced
2 tablespoons rice vinegar
1 garlic clove, minced

1. In a large bowl, toss together the green and red cabbage, carrots, and scallions. 2. In a small bowl, whisk together the oil, vinegar, honey, garlic, and salt. 3. Pour the dressing over the veggies and mix to thoroughly combine. 4. Serve immediately, or cover and chill for several hours before serving.

**Per Serving**

Calories: 80 | fat: 5g | protein: 1g | carbs: 10g | sugars: 6g | fiber: 3g | sodium: 126mg

# Winter Chicken and Citrus Salad

## Prep time: 10 minutes | Cook time: 0 minutes | Serves 4

4 cups baby spinach

1 tablespoon freshly squeezed lemon juice

Freshly ground black pepper

2 mandarin oranges, peeled and sectioned

¼ cup sliced almonds

2 tablespoons extra-virgin olive oil

⅛ teaspoon salt

2 cups chopped cooked chicken

½ peeled grapefruit, sectioned

1. In a large mixing bowl, toss the spinach with the olive oil, lemon juice, salt, and pepper. 2. Add the chicken, oranges, grapefruit, and almonds to the bowl. Toss gently. 3. Arrange on 4 plates and serve.

**Per Serving**

Calories: 249 | fat: 12g | protein: 24g | carbs: 11g | sugars: 7g | fiber: 3g | sodium: 135mg

# Mediterranean Vegetable Salad

## Prep time: 10 minutes | Cook time: 0 minutes | Serves 6

⅓ cup tarragon vinegar or white wine vinegar

2 tablespoons chopped fresh or 2 teaspoons dried oregano leaves

½ teaspoon ground mustard

2 cloves garlic, finely chopped

2 large yellow bell peppers, sliced into thin rings

½ cup crumbled feta cheese (2 ounces)

Kalamata olives, if desired

2 tablespoons canola or soybean oil

½ teaspoon sugar

½ teaspoon salt

½ teaspoon pepper

3 large tomatoes, sliced

6 ounces fresh spinach leaves (from 10-ounce bag), stems removed (about 1 cup)

1. In small bowl, mix vinegar, oil, oregano, sugar, salt, mustard, pepper and garlic. In glass or plastic container, place tomatoes and bell peppers. Pour vinegar mixture over vegetables. Cover and refrigerate at least 1 hour to blend flavors. 2. Line serving platter with spinach. Drain vegetables; place on spinach. Sprinkle with cheese; garnish with olives.

**Per Serving**

Calorie: 110 | fat: 8g | protein: 3g | carbs: 8g | sugars: 6g | fiber: 1g | sodium: 340mg

# Crunchy Pecan Tuna Salad

## Prep time: 20 minutes | Cook time: 0 minutes | Serves 1

½ medium apple, finely chopped

¼ large red onion, finely chopped

¼ cup canned navy beans, drained, rinsed, and mashed

½ tablespoon Dijon mustard

Black pepper, as needed

2 medium ribs celery, finely chopped

2 tablespoons coarsely chopped pecans

2 ounces canned tuna packed in water, drained and rinsed

1 tablespoon mayonnaise (see Tip)

1 tablespoon fresh lemon juice

1. In a large bowl, combine the apple, celery, onion, pecans, beans, and tuna. 2. In a small bowl, mix together the mayonnaise, mustard, lemon juice, and black pepper. Add the mayonnaise mixture to the tuna mixture and stir until the tuna salad is evenly combined. 3. Serve the tuna salad immediately, or refrigerate the tuna salad for 2 to 3 hours or overnight to chill it and allow the flavors to meld.

**Per Serving**

Calorie: 197 | fat: 11g | protein: 11g | carbs: 16g | sugars: 7g | fiber: 5g | sodium: 179mg

# Greek Rice Salad

**Prep time: 10 minutes | Cook time: 0 minutes | Serves 4**

3 tablespoons fresh lemon juice

1 tablespoon red wine vinegar

1 teaspoon Dijon mustard

½–1 teaspoon grated fresh garlic

4 cups cooked brown rice

1 cup sliced grape or cherry tomatoes or chopped tomatoes (can substitute chopped red pepper)

2 tablespoons chopped fresh dill

1½ tablespoons coconut nectar or pure maple syrup

1 teaspoon sea salt

¼ teaspoon allspice

Freshly ground black pepper to taste (optional)

1 cup chopped cucumber (seeds removed, if you prefer)

½ cup sliced kalamata olives

½ tablespoon chopped fresh oregano

1. In a large bowl, whisk together the lemon juice, nectar or syrup, vinegar, salt, mustard, allspice, garlic, and pepper (if using). Add the rice, cucumber, tomatoes, olives, oregano, and dill, and stir to combine. Taste, and add extra salt or lemon juice, if desired. Serve as a side or as a hearty lunch over greens.

**Per Serving**
Calorie: 306 | fat: 4g | protein: 6g | carbs: 62g | sugars: 7g | fiber: 5g | sodium: 751mg

# Triple-Berry and Jicama Spinach Salad

**Prep time: 30 minutes | Cook time: 0 minutes | Serves 6**

**Dressing**

¼ cup fresh raspberries

2 tablespoons canola oil

2 medium jalapeño chiles, seeded, finely chopped (2 tablespoons)

1 small clove garlic, crushed

**Salad**

1 bag (6 ounces) fresh baby spinach leaves

1 cup fresh blackberries

1 cup sliced fresh strawberries

3 tablespoons hot pepper jelly

2 tablespoons raspberry vinegar or red wine vinegar

2 teaspoons finely chopped shallot

¼ teaspoon salt

1 cup bite-size strips (1x¼x¼ inch) peeled jicama

1 cup fresh raspberries

1. In small food processor or blender, combine all dressing ingredients; process until smooth. 2. In large bowl, toss spinach and ¼ cup of the dressing. On 6 serving plates, arrange salad. To serve, top each salad with jicama, blackberries, raspberries, strawberries and drizzle with scant 1 tablespoon of remaining dressing.

**Per Serving**
Calorie: 120 | fat: 5g | protein: 2g | carbs: 18g | sugars: 9g | fiber: 5g | sodium: 125mg

# Five-Layer Salad

**Prep time: 10 minutes | Cook time: 6 minutes | Serves 6**

1 cup frozen sweet peas

⅓ cup plain fat-free yogurt

1 tablespoon cider vinegar

2 teaspoons sugar

3 cups coleslaw mix (shredded cabbage and carrots; from 16-ounce bag)

1 tablespoon water

¼ cup reduced-fat mayonnaise (do not use salad dressing)

½ teaspoon salt

1 cup shredded carrots (2 medium)

1 cup halved cherry tomatoes

1. In small microwavable bowl, place peas and water. Cover with microwavable plastic wrap, folding back one edge ¼ inch to vent steam. Microwave on High 4 to 6 minutes, stirring after 2 minutes, until tender; drain. Let stand until cool. 2. Meanwhile, in small bowl, mix yogurt, mayonnaise, vinegar, sugar and salt. 3. In 1½- or 2-quart glass bowl, layer coleslaw mix, carrots, tomatoes and peas. Spread mayonnaise mixture over top. Refrigerate 15 minutes. Toss gently before serving.

**Per Serving**
Calorie: 100 | fat: 3.5g | protein: 3g | carbs: 13g | sugars: 7g | fiber: 3g | sodium: 330mg

# Mediterranean Pasta Salad with Goat Cheese

## Prep time: 25 minutes | Cook time: 0 minutes | Serves 4

½ cup grape tomatoes, sliced in half lengthwise
½ medium red onion, sliced into thin strips
1 cup broccoli florets
¼ cup olive oil
½ teaspoon black pepper
½ teaspoon garlic powder
½ cup shaved Parmesan cheese

1 medium red bell pepper, coarsely chopped
1 medium zucchini, coarsely chopped
½ cup oil-packed artichoke hearts, drained
½ teaspoon sea salt
1 tablespoon dried oregano
4 ounces crumbled goat cheese
8 ounces lentil or chickpea penne pasta, cooked, rinsed, and drained

1. In a large bowl, combine the tomatoes, bell pepper, onion, zucchini, broccoli, artichoke hearts, oil, sea salt, black pepper, oregano, garlic powder, goat cheese, and Parmesan cheese. Gently mix everything together to combine and coat all of the ingredients with the oil. 2. Add the pasta to the bowl and stir to combine. 3. Let the pasta salad rest for 1 to 2 hours in the refrigerator to marinate it, or serve the pasta salad immediately if desired.

**Per Serving**
Calorie: 477 | fat: 24g | protein: 23g | carbs: 41g | sugars: 6g | fiber: 6g | sodium: 706mg

# Moroccan Carrot Salad

## Prep time: 15 minutes | Cook time: 0 minutes | Serves 5

**Dressing**
¼ cup orange juice
1 teaspoon orange peel
1 teaspoon paprika
⅛ to ¼ teaspoon ground red pepper (cayenne)
**Salad**
1 bag (10 ounces) julienne (matchstick-cut) carrots (5 cups)
1 can (15 ounces) chickpeas (garbanzo beans), drained, rinsed
¼ cup golden raisins
3 tablespoons salted roasted whole almonds, coarsely chopped
¼ cup coarsely chopped fresh cilantro or parsley

2 tablespoons olive oil
1 teaspoon ground cumin
¼ teaspoon salt
⅛ teaspoon ground cinnamon

1. In small bowl, combine all dressing ingredients with whisk until blended; set aside. 2. In large bowl, combine carrots, chickpeas and raisins; toss to combine. Add dressing; mix thoroughly. Cover and refrigerate at least 2 hours or overnight, stirring occasionally. Just before serving, sprinkle with almonds and cilantro.

**Per Serving**
Calorie: 310 | fat: 11g | protein: 10g | carbs: 44g | sugars: 12g | fiber: 10g | sodium: 230mg

# Celery and Apple Salad with Cider Vinaigrette

## Prep time: 20 minutes | Cook time: 0 minutes | Serves 4

### Dressing
2 tablespoons apple cider or apple juice

2 teaspoons canola oil

½ teaspoon Dijon mustard

½ teaspoon salt

1 tablespoon cider vinegar

2 teaspoons finely chopped shallots

½ teaspoon honey

### Salad
2 cups chopped romaine lettuce

½ medium apple, unpeeled, sliced very thin (about 1 cup)

2 tablespoons crumbled blue cheese

2 cups diagonally sliced celery

⅓ cup sweetened dried cranberries

2 tablespoons chopped walnuts

1. In small bowl, beat all dressing ingredients with whisk until blended; set aside. 2. In medium bowl, place lettuce, celery, apple and cranberries; toss with dressing. To serve, arrange salad on 4 plates. Sprinkle with walnuts and blue cheese. Serve immediately.

### Per Serving
Calorie: 130 | fat: 6g | protein: 2g | carbs: 17g | sugars: 13g | fiber: 3g | sodium: 410mg

# Thai Broccoli Slaw

## Prep time: 20 minutes | Cook time: 0 minutes | Serves 8

### Dressing
2 tablespoons reduced-fat creamy peanut butter

1 tablespoon rice vinegar

1½ teaspoons reduced-sodium soy sauce

1 tablespoon grated gingerroot

1 tablespoon orange marmalade

¼ to ½ teaspoon chili garlic sauce

### Slaw
3 cups broccoli slaw mix (from 10-ounce bag)

½ cup julienne (matchstick-cut) carrots

2 tablespoons chopped fresh cilantro

½ cup bite-size thin strips red bell pepper

½ cup shredded red cabbage

1. In small bowl, combine all dressing ingredients. Beat with whisk, until blended. 2. In large bowl, toss all slaw ingredients. Pour dressing over slaw mixture; toss until coated. Cover and refrigerate at least 1 hour to blend flavors but no longer than 6 hours, tossing occasionally to blend dressing from bottom of bowl back into slaw mixture.

### Per Serving
Calorie: 50 | fat: 1.5g | protein: 2g | carbs: 7g | sugars: 3g | fiber: 1g | sodium: 75mg

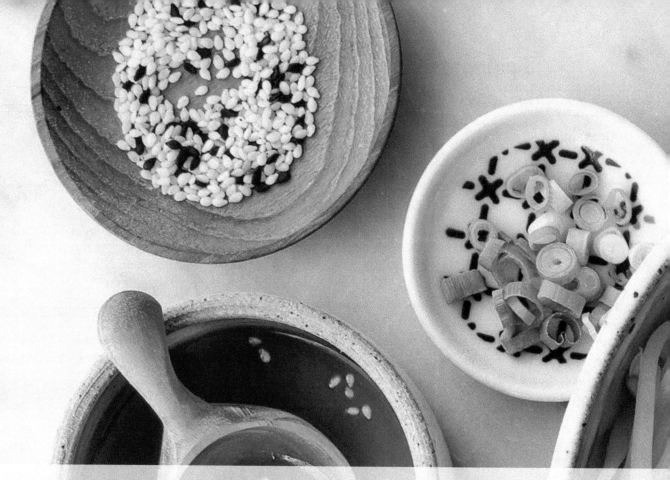

# Chapter 7    Staples, Sauces, Dips, and Dressings

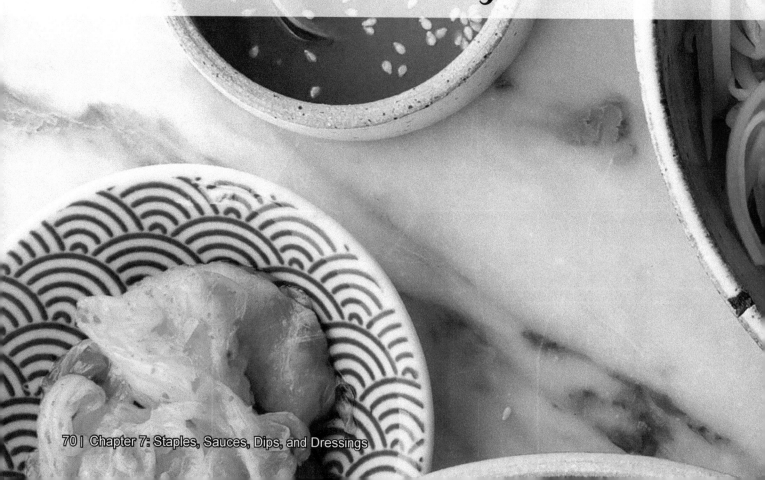

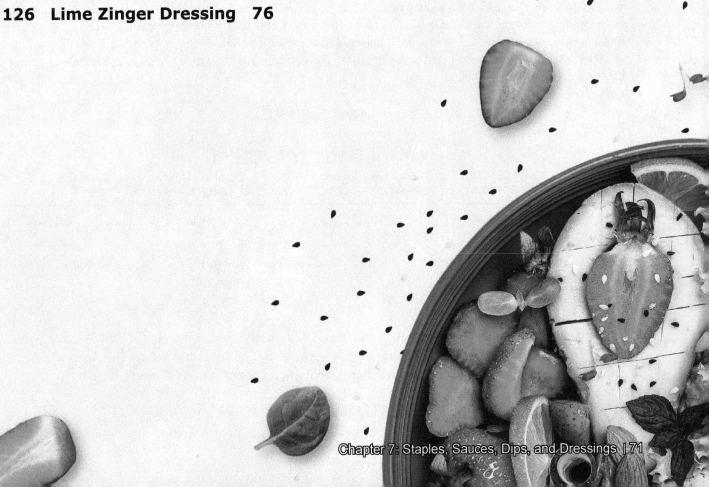

# Mango-Hemp Dressing

## Prep time: 10 minutes | Cook time: 0 minutes | Serves 8

¾ cup mango chunks, fresh or frozen
2 tablespoons freshly squeezed lime juice or red wine vinegar
½ teaspoon Dijon mustard
Freshly ground black pepper to taste
1–2 tablespoons coconut nectar or pure maple syrup

2 tablespoons hemp seeds
½ tablespoon chopped shallots or 1 tablespoon of the whitish portion of a green onion
½ teaspoon sea salt
¼ cup + 2–3 teaspoons water (optional)

1. In a blender, combine the mango, hemp, lime juice or vinegar, shallots or green onion, mustard, salt, pepper, ¼ cup of the water, and 1 tablespoon of the nectar or syrup. Puree until very smooth. Taste, and add the remaining 2 to 3 tablespoons water to thin (if desired) and the remaining 1 tablespoon nectar or syrup, to taste.

**Per Serving**

Calorie: 31 | fat: 1g | protein: 1g | carbs: 5g | sugars: 4g | fiber: 1g | sodium: 155mg

# Spiced Sweet Potato Hummus

## Prep time: 10 minutes | Cook time: 0 minutes | Serves 4

1 can (15 ounces) kidney beans, rinsed (about 1¾ cups)
2 tablespoons tahini
¼ teaspoon cinnamon
4–4½ tablespoons freshly squeezed lime juice
1–3 tablespoons water

1 can (15 ounces) chickpeas, rinsed (about 1¾ cups)
1 cup cooked and peeled orange sweet potato
1 teaspoon sea salt
1 medium or large clove garlic, sliced or quartered
½–1 teaspoon chili powder (adjust to taste)
Fresh cilantro or parsley (optional)

1. In a food procesor, combine the kidney beans, chickpeas, sweet potato, tahini, salt, cinnamon, garlic, lime juice, ½ teaspoon of the chili powder, and 1 tablespoon of the water. Puree until smooth, gradually adding the remaining 2 tablespoons of water if needed to thin the hummus and scraping down the sides of the bowl as needed. Add the fresh cilantro or parsley (if using), and puree briefly to incorporate. Season with additional salt and the remaining ½ teaspoon chili powder, if desired.

**Per Serving**

Calorie: 275 | fat: 7g | protein: 13g | carbs: 43g | sugars: 9g | fiber: 11g | sodium: 914mg

# Lentil Baba Ghanoush

## Prep time: 10 minutes | Cook time: 0 minutes | Serves 4

2 cups cooked brown lentils
1 large clove garlic
Rounded ¼ teaspoon smoked paprika
2 tablespoons tahini
1–4 tablespoons water (as needed to smooth)

1½ tablespoons chopped fresh oregano leaves
½ teaspoon sea salt
½ teaspoon lemon zest
3½–4 tablespoons lemon juice
Drizzle of tamari (optional)

1. In a food processor, combine the lentils, oregano, garlic, salt, paprika, lemon zest, tahini, and 3½ tablespoons of the lemon juice. Puree until smooth, adding the water as needed, 1 tablespoon at a time. Taste, and add the remaining ½ tablespoon lemon juice, if desired. Serve, adding a drizzle of tamari (if using).

**Per Serving**

Calorie: 165 | fat: 5g | protein: 10g | carbs: 23g | sugars: 1g | fiber: 7g | sodium: 307mg

# Asian-Fusion Hummus

## Prep time: 10 minutes | Cook time: 0 minutes | Serves 8

4 cups cooked chickpeas (rinse and drain if using canned)
1 medium-large clove garlic, sliced
1 pitted date
¼–⅓ cup freshly squeezed lime juice
Sea salt to taste

2 tablespoons orange juice
3 tablespoons peanut butter or tahini
1 tablespoon grated fresh ginger
3 tablespoons tamari
2–4 tablespoons water
⅛ teaspoon crushed red-pepper flakes (optional)

1. In a food processor, combine the chickpeas, orange juice, peanut butter or tahini, garlic, ginger, date, tamari, ¼ cup of the lime juice, and 2 tablespoons of the water. Puree until very smooth. Taste, and add the remaining lime juice for more tang, if you like, and the additional 2 tablespoons of water, if needed to achieve a smoother texture. Puree until well combined. Add salt to taste and the red-pepper flakes (if using).

**Per Serving**

Calorie: 182 | fat: 5g | protein: 9g | carbs: 26g | sugars: 6g | fiber: 7g | sodium: 555mg

# Punchy Mustard Vinaigrette

## Prep time: 5 minutes | Cook time: 0 minutes | Serves 6

¼ cup apple cider vinegar or rice vinegar
1½ tablespoons yellow or Dijon mustard
½ tablespoon ground chia
⅛ teaspoon sea salt

2 tablespoons tamari
2½ tablespoons coconut nectar or pure maple syrup
Freshly ground black pepper to taste

1. In a blender, combine the vinegar, tamari, mustard, nectar or syrup, chia, pepper, and salt. Puree until fully incorporated. Taste, and add extra mustard if you love it! Season to taste with additional salt and pepper, if desired. Serve immediately or refrigerate. Dressing will keep for at least a week in the fridge.

**Per Serving**

Calorie: 33 | fat: 0g | protein: 1g | carbs: 7g | sugars: 5g | fiber: 1g | sodium: 428mg

# Irresistible White Bean Dip

## Prep time: 5 minutes | Cook time: 0 minutes | Serves 4

1 can (15 ounces) white beans, rinsed and drained
2 teaspoons miso
¼ teaspoon black salt
1 tablespoon nutritional yeast
¼–½ teaspoon pure maple syrup (optional)

2 tablespoons lemon juice
Scant ½ teaspoon sea salt
1 tablespoon tahini
1 clove garlic (or to taste)
1–1½ tablespoons water

1. In a small food processor or high-powered blender, combine the beans, lemon juice, miso, sea salt, black salt, tahini, yeast, garlic, syrup (if using), and 1 tablespoon of the water. Puree, adding the additional ½ tablespoon water if needed. (Just don't add too much; the dip should be thick.) Taste, and season with extra lemon, salt, or garlic, if desired.

**Per Serving**

Calorie: 139 | fat: 3g | protein: 9g | carbs: 21g | sugars: 1g | fiber: 6g | sodium: 638mg

# Chocolate Orange Dip

## Prep time: 10 minutes | Cook time: 0 minutes | Serves 4

1 cup (packed) pitted dates
2 tablespoons almond or cashew butter (or
1½ tablespoons softened coconut butter, for nut-free)
¼ teaspoon sea salt
¼ cup cocoa powder
2 tablespoons mini chocolate chips (optional)

1 can (15 ounces) white beans, drained and rinsed
1 teaspoon orange zest
¼ teaspoon vanilla powder or 1 teaspoon
pure vanilla extract
1–2 tablespoons coconut nectar or pure
maple syrup (optional)

1. In a food processor, combine the dates, orange juice, white beans, nut butter, orange zest, vanilla powder or extract, and salt. Puree until smooth. Add the cocoa powder and puree again. Taste, and add the nectar or syrup to sweeten, if desired. Pulse in or garnish with the chocolate chips (if using). Serve or transfer to an airtight container and refrigerate for up to 6 days.

**Per Serving**
Calorie: 275 | fat: 6g | protein: 11g | carbs: 53g | sugars: 26g | fiber: 10g | sodium: 279mg

# Beet-Yogurt Dip

## Prep time: 10 minutes | Cook time: 45 to 60 minutes | Serves 6

½ pound red beets
1 tablespoon extra-virgin olive oil
1 garlic clove, peeled
½ teaspoon onion powder

½ cup plain nonfat Greek yogurt
1 tablespoon freshly squeezed lemon juice
1 teaspoon minced fresh thyme
¼ teaspoon salt

1. Preheat the oven to 375°F. 2. Wrap the beets in aluminum foil and bake for 45 to 60 minutes until the beets are tender when pierced with a fork. Set aside and let cool for at least 10 minutes. Using your hands, remove the skins and transfer the beets to a blender. 3. To the blender jar, add the yogurt, olive oil, lemon juice, garlic, thyme, onion powder, and salt. Process until smooth. Chill for 1 hour before serving.

**Per Serving**
Calories: 49 | fat: 2g | protein: 3g | carbs: 5g | sugars: 3g | fiber: 1g | sodium: 121mg

# Green Chickpea Hummus

## Prep time: 5 minutes | Cook time: 0 minutes | Serves 6

2 cups frozen green chickpeas
¼ cup lemon juice
⅓ cup fresh basil leaves
1 tablespoon tahini
½ teaspoon ground cumin
½ teaspoon lemon zest (optional)

1 can (15 ounces) white beans, rinsed and drained
1 large clove garlic (or more to taste)
⅓ cup fresh parsley leaves
1 teaspoon sea salt
1–2 tablespoons water (optional)

1. Add the chickpeas to a pot of boiling water and cook for just a minute to bring out their vibrant green color. Remove, run under cold water to stop the cooking process, and drain. In a food processor, combine the chickpeas, beans, lemon juice, garlic, basil, parsley, tahini, salt, and cumin. Puree until smooth, scraping down the bowl as needed. Add the water if desired to thin or help the pureeing process. Add the lemon zest, if desired, and season to taste. Serve.

**Per Serving**
Calorie: 176 | fat: 3g | protein: 10g | carbs: 29g | sugars: 3g | fiber: 8g | sodium: 477mg

# Salsa Makeover

## Prep time: 5 minutes | Cook time: 0 minutes | Serves 5

1 cup store-bought fresh or jarred salsa
½ cup diced red pepper
½ tablespoon lime juice
Few tablespoons chopped fresh cilantro
or fresh parsley (optional)

⅔ cup small cubes ripe avocado (about 1 avocado)
½ cup frozen corn kernels, thawed
in a bowl of boiled water
Sea salt
Freshly ground pepper to taste (optional)

1. In a large bowl, combine the salsa, avocado, red pepper, corn, lime juice, and cilantro or parsley (if using). Mix together. Season to taste with salt and pepper, if using.

**Per Serving**

Calorie: 78 | fat: 4g | protein: 2g | carbs: 10g | sugars: 3g | fiber: 3g | sodium: 368mg

# Balsamic Drizzle

## Prep time: 5 minutes | Cook time: 30 minutes | Serves 5

½ cup balsamic vinegar
Pinch or two of sea salt

2 tablespoons coconut nectar

1. In a saucepan over medium-high heat, combine the vinegar, coconut nectar, and salt. Bring the mixture to a boil, then reduce the heat to medium-low. Let the mixture gently boil for 25 to 30 minutes, or until it has thickened and reduced in volume. If you'd like it thicker, let it cook for a few additional minutes. Remove from the heat and let it cool. (It will thicken a little more with cooling.) Leftovers can be stored in a jar or bottle in the fridge.

**Per Serving**

Calorie: 40 | fat: 2g | protein: 0g | carbs: 9g | sugars: 8g | fiber: 3g | sodium: 62mg

# Fresh Salsa

## Prep time: 10 minutes | Cook time: 0 minutes | Serves 4

2 cups chopped tomatoes
¼ cup minced red, yellow, or orange bell pepper
1 large clove garlic, minced or grated
1 tablespoon lime juice
½ teaspoon cumin (optional)
Freshly ground black pepper to taste

¼ cup minced onion or ⅓ cup chopped green onion
1 small jalapeño pepper, seeded and minced,
wear plastic gloves when handling
½ teaspoon sea salt
⅛ teaspoon allspice
¼ cup minced cilantro (optional)

1. In a large bowl, combine the tomatoes, onion, bell pepper, jalapeño pepper, garlic, lime juice, salt, cumin (if using), allspice, black pepper, and cilantro (if using). Stir to combine. Taste, and add extra salt or spices as desired. Serve or refrigerate in an airtight container until ready to use (within 2 to 3 days).

**Per Serving**

Calorie: 27 | fat: 0g | protein: 1g | carbs: 6g | sugars: 3g | fiber: 2g | sodium: 301mg

# Lightened Tahini Sauce

## Prep time: 5 minutes | Cook time: 0 minutes | Serves 8

⅓ cup tahini
3 tablespoons lemon juice
1–2 teaspoons coconut nectar (optional)
Sea salt

⅓ cup unsweetened applesauce
2 tablespoons tamari
2–4 tablespoons water
Freshly ground black pepper

1. In a blender (or using an immersion blender and a deep cup), combine the tahini, applesauce, lemon juice, tamari, nectar (if using), 2 tablespoons of the water, and salt and pepper to taste. Puree until smooth. Add the additional 1 to 2 tablespoons water if desired to thin the sauce. Season to taste, and serve.
**Per Serving**
Calorie: 68 | fat: 5g | protein: 2g | carbs: 4g | sugars: 1g | fiber: 1g | sodium: 559mg

# Fresh Tomato Salsa

## Prep time: 10 minutes | Cook time: 0 minutes | Serves 6

2 or 3 medium, ripe tomatoes, diced
1 serrano pepper, seeded and minced
¼ cup minced fresh cilantro

½ red onion, minced
Juice of 1 lime
¼ teaspoon salt

1. In a small bowl, combine the tomatoes, onion, serrano pepper, lime juice, cilantro, and salt, and mix well. Taste and season with additional salt as needed. 2. Serve immediately, or transfer to an airtight container and refrigerate for up to 3 days.
**Per Serving**
Calorie: 18 | fat: 0g | protein: 1g | carbs: 4g | sugars: 1g | fiber: 1g | sodium: 84mg

# Lime Zinger Dressing

## Prep time: 5 minutes | Cook time: 0 minutes | Serves 4

¼ cup freshly squeezed lime juice
½ tablespoon ground chia seeds
½ teaspoon ground cumin
Pinch of allspice
Freshly ground black pepper to taste

3 tablespoons coconut nectar
½ tablespoon Dijon mustard
¼ teaspoon cinnamon
½ teaspoon sea salt
1 tablespoon water (optional)

1. In a blender, combine the lime juice, nectar, chia seeds, mustard, cumin, cinnamon, allspice, salt, and pepper. Puree until smooth. Add the water if desired to thin. Transfer to a jar or other airtight container and refrigerate for up to a week.
**Per Serving**
Calorie: 52 | fat: 1g | protein: 0g | carbs: 12g | sugars: 9g | fiber: 1g | sodium: 340mg

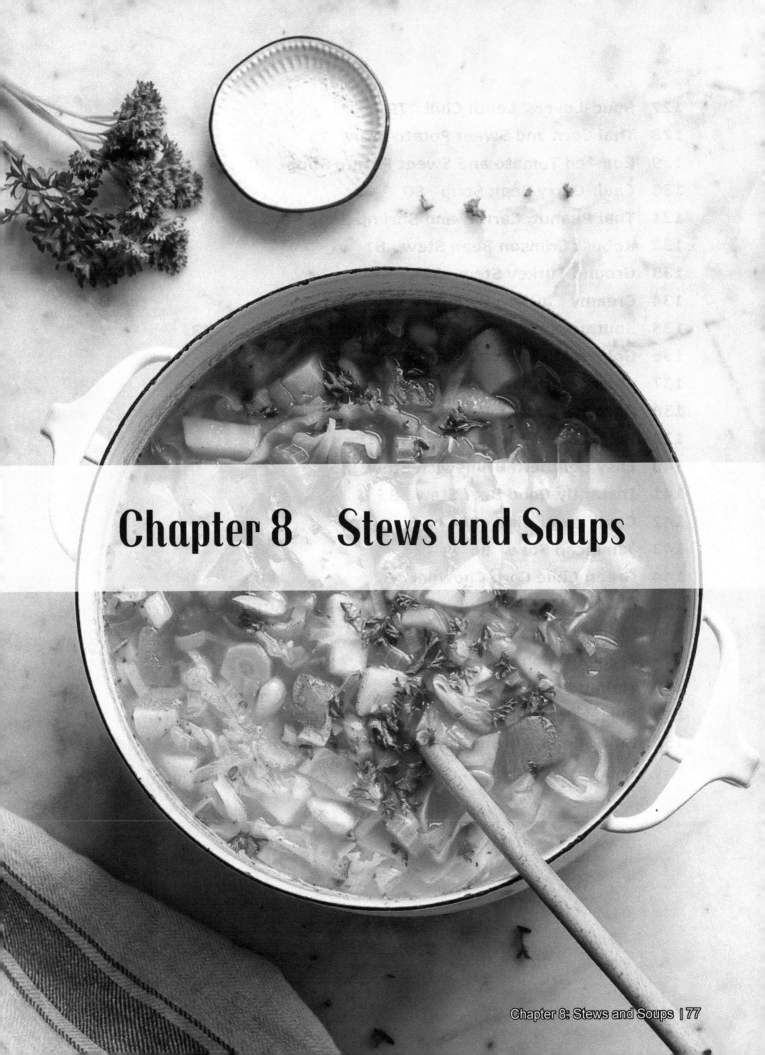

# Chapter 8     Stews and Soups

# Spud-Lovers' Lentil Chili

## Prep time: 10 minutes | Cook time: 50 minutes | Serves 6

1½ cups onions, finely chopped
2 cups cubed sweet potatoes (can use frozen)
1¼ teaspoons sea salt
1 teaspoon dried oregano
1 teaspoon ground cumin
2 tablespoons finely chopped pitted dates
1 cup dried red lentils
1 can (28 ounces) crushed tomatoes
Lime wedges

2 cups cubed red or yellow potatoes (not russet)
3–4 large cloves garlic, minced
1 tablespoon chili powder
1 teaspoon paprika or smoked paprika
½ teaspoon cinnamon
2–5 tablespoons + 3½ cups water
1 cup dried green lentils
2–3 tablespoons freshly squeezed lime juice

1. In a large pot over medium heat, combine the onions, potatoes, sweet potatoes, garlic, salt, chili powder, oregano, paprika, cumin, cinnamon, dates, and 2 to 3 tablespoons of the water, and stir. Cover and cook for 6 to 8 minutes, stirring occasionally. Reduce the heat if the mixture is sticking to the bottom of the pot, and add 1 to 2 tablespoons of water. Rinse the red and green lentils. Add the lentils, tomatoes, and remaining 3½ cups water to the pot, and stir to combine. Increase the heat to bring to a boil. Reduce the heat to low, cover, and simmer for 40 minutes or longer, until the green lentils are fully cooked through and softened. Stir in the lime juice (adjusting to taste), and serve portions with lime wedges.

**Per Serving**

Calorie: 337 | fat: 2g | protein: 19g | carbs: 66g | sugars: 11g | fiber: 17g | sodium: 698mg

# Thai Corn and Sweet Potato Stew

## Prep time: 10 minutes | Cook time: 20 minutes | Serves 4

1 small can (5.5 ounces) light coconut milk
½ cup chopped celery
¾–1 teaspoon sea salt
1½ tablespoons Thai yellow or red curry paste
1½ cups chopped red bell pepper
2½ tablespoons freshly squeezed lime juice
4–5 cups baby spinach leaves
Lime wedges (optional)

1 cup chopped onion
2 cups cubed sweet potato (can use frozen)
2 cups water
1½ cups frozen corn kernels
1 package (12–14 ounces) tofu, cut into cubes,
or 1 can (14 ounces) black beans, rinsed and drained
⅓–½ cup fresh cilantro or Thai basil, chopped

1. In a soup pot over high heat, warm 2 tablespoons of the coconut milk. Add the onion, celery, sweet potato, and ¾ teaspoon of the salt, and sauté for 4 to 5 minutes. Add the water, Thai paste, and remaining coconut milk. Increase the heat to high to bring to a boil. Cover and reduce the heat to medium-low, and let the mixture simmer for 8 to 10 minutes, or until the sweet potato has softened. Turn off the heat, and use an immersion blender to puree the soup base. Add the corn, bell pepper, and tofu or beans, and turn the heat to medium-low. Cover and cook for 3 to 4 minutes to heat through. Add the lime juice, spinach, and cilantro or basil, and stir until the spinach has just wilted. Taste, and season with the remaining ¼ teaspoon salt, if desired. Serve with the lime wedges (if using).

**Per Serving**

Calorie: 223 | fat: 7g | protein: 10g | carbs: 36g | sugars: 11g | fiber: 6g | sodium: 723mg

# Roasted Tomato and Sweet Potato Soup

## Prep time: 10 minutes | Cook time: 40 to 50 minutes | Serves 4

1½ cups onions, finely chopped

2 cups cubed sweet potatoes (can use frozen)

1¼ teaspoons sea salt

4 cups cubed sweet potato (roughly 1–1¼ pounds before peeling)

1½ teaspoons dried basil

1 tablespoon balsamic vinegar

Freshly ground black pepper to taste

2¼–2½ cups water

2 cups cubed red or yellow potatoes (not russet)

3–4 large cloves garlic, minced

1½ cups peeled, quartered onion (roughly 1 large onion)

4 cups (about 1½ pounds) quartered Roma or other tomatoes, juices squeezed out

1½ teaspoons dried oregano

1 teaspoon blackstrap molasses

1⅛ teaspoons sea salt

¼ cup chopped fresh basil (optional)

1. Preheat the oven to 450°F. 2. In a large baking dish, combine the onion, sweet potato, tomatoes, basil, oregano, vinegar, molasses, pepper, and 1 teaspoon of the salt. Cook for 40 to 50 minutes, stirring a couple of times, until the sweet potatoes are softened and the mixture is becoming caramelized. Transfer the vegetables and any juices they've released in the pan to a medium soup pot, add 2¼ cups of the water and the remaining ⅛ teaspoon salt, and use an immersion blender to puree. (Alternatively, you can transfer everything to a blender to puree.) Blend to the desired smoothness, using the additional ¼ cup water if needed. Stir in fresh basil, if using, and serve.

**Per Serving**

Calorie: 152 | fat: 0.4g | protein: 4g | carbs: 35g | sugars: 14g | fiber: 5g | sodium: 648mg

# Cauli-Curry Bean Soup

## Prep time: 10 minutes | Cook time: 25 minutes | Serves 8

2 cups chopped onion

1½ tablespoons curry powder (or to taste; use more if you really love curry)

1 teaspoon mustard seeds

1 teaspoon ground turmeric

⅛ teaspoon ground cinnamon

3–4 cups cauliflower florets

1 can (15 ounces) adzuki or black beans, rinsed and drained

1 tablespoon grated fresh ginger

1½ cups chopped carrot or sweet potato

1¼ teaspoons sea salt

Freshly ground black pepper to taste

1 teaspoon ground cumin

¼ teaspoon ground cardamom

4–5 tablespoons + 4 cups water

1 can (15 ounces) chickpeas, rinsed and drained

1 cup dried red lentils

1 can (28 ounces) crushed tomatoes

1–2 teaspoons pure maple syrup (optional)

1. In a large pot over medium-high heat, combine the onion, carrot or sweet potato, curry powder, salt, pepper, mustard seeds, cumin, turmeric, cardamom, cinnamon, and 3 tablespoons of the water. Stir, cover, and cook for 4 to 5 minutes, stirring occasionally. (Add another 1 to 2 tablespoons of water if needed to keep the vegetables and spices from sticking.) Add the cauliflower, chickpeas, beans, lentils, tomatoes, and remaining 4 cups water. Stir and increase the heat to high to bring to a boil. Reduce the heat to low, cover, and simmer for 15 to 20 minutes. Stir in the ginger and syrup (if using). Season to taste, and serve.

**Per Serving**

Calorie: 226 | fat: 2g | protein: 14g | carbs: 42g | sugars: 7g | fiber: 13g | sodium: 577mg

# Thai Peanut, Carrot, and Shrimp Soup

## Prep time: 10 minutes | Cook time: 10 minutes | Serves 4

| | |
|---|---|
| 1 tablespoon coconut oil | 1 tablespoon Thai red curry paste |
| ½ onion, sliced | 3 garlic cloves, minced |
| 2 cups chopped carrots | ½ cup whole unsalted peanuts |
| 4 cups low-sodium vegetable broth | ½ cup unsweetened plain almond milk |
| ½ pound shrimp, peeled and deveined | Minced fresh cilantro, for garnish |

1. In a large pan, heat the oil over medium-high heat until shimmering. 2. Add the curry paste and cook, stirring constantly, for 1 minute. Add the onion, garlic, carrots, and peanuts to the pan, and continue to cook for 2 to 3 minutes until the onion begins to soften. 3. Add the broth and bring to a boil. Reduce the heat to low and simmer for 5 to 6 minutes until the carrots are tender. 4. Using an immersion blender or in a blender, purée the soup until smooth and return it to the pot. With the heat still on low, add the almond milk and stir to combine. Add the shrimp to the pot and cook for 2 to 3 minutes until cooked through. 5. Garnish with cilantro and serve.

**Per Serving**

Calories: 237 | fat: 14g | protein: 14g | carbs: 17g | sugars: 6g | fiber: 5g | sodium: 619mg

# Robust Crimson Bean Stew

## Prep time: 10 minutes | Cook time: 20 minutes | Serves 4

| | |
|---|---|
| 1 cup chopped red onion | 2 teaspoons dried oregano |
| 1 teaspoon dried rosemary | 1 teaspoon Dijon mustard |
| Freshly ground black pepper to taste | 2 tablespoons + 2½ cups water |
| 2 cups cubed yellow or red potatoes | ½ cup dry black beluga or French lentils |
| ½ cup uncooked brown or red rice | (can substitute green or brown lentils) |
| (can substitute quinoa) | 3 cloves minced or grated garlic |
| 1 can (28 ounces) crushed tomatoes | 1 can (15 ounces) adzuki, black, or kidney beans, |
| 1–1½ cups chopped red peppers | rinsed and drained |
| 2 tablespoons vegan Worcestershire sauce | ¼ teaspoon sea salt |

1. In an instant pot set on the sauté function, combine the onion, oregano, rosemary, mustard, black pepper, and 2 tablespoons of the water. Cook for 3 to 4 minutes. Turn off the sauté function and stir in the potatoes, lentils, rice, garlic, tomatoes, beans, and remaining 2½ cups water. Cook on high pressure for 15 minutes, and either release the pressure manually or let it naturally release. Add the red peppers, Worcestershire sauce, and salt to the instant pot. Stir, replace the cover, and let sit for 5 to 8 minutes. Taste, season as desired, and serve.

**Per Serving**

Calorie: 596 | fat: 2g | protein: 29g | carbs: 120g | sugars: 11g | fiber: 28g | sodium: 523mg

# Ground Turkey Stew

**Prep time: 5 minutes | Cook time: 25 minutes | Serves 5**

| | |
|---|---|
| 1 tablespoon olive oil | 1 onion, chopped |
| 1 pound ground turkey | ½ teaspoon garlic powder |
| 1 teaspoon chili powder | ¾ teaspoon cumin |
| 2 teaspoons coriander | 1 teaspoon dried oregano |
| ½ teaspoon salt | 1 green pepper, chopped |
| 1 red pepper, chopped | 1 tomato, chopped |
| 1½ cups reduced-sodium tomato sauce | 1 tablespoon low-sodium soy sauce |
| 1 cup water | 2 handfuls cilantro, chopped |
| 15-ounce can reduced-salt black beans | |

1. Press the Sauté function on the control panel of the Instant Pot. 2. Add the olive oil to the inner pot and let it get hot. Add onion and sauté for a few minutes, or until light golden. 3. Add ground turkey. Break the ground meat using a wooden spoon to avoid formation of lumps. Sauté for a few minutes, until the pink color has faded. 4. Add garlic powder, chili powder, cumin, coriander, dried oregano, and salt. Combine well. Add green pepper, red pepper, and chopped tomato. Combine well. 5. Add tomato sauce, soy sauce, and water; combine well. 6. Close and secure the lid. Click on the Cancel key to cancel the Sauté mode. Make sure the pressure release valve on the lid is in the sealing position. 7. Click on Manual function first and then select high pressure. Click the + button and set the time to 15 minutes. 8. You can either have the steam release naturally (it will take around 20 minutes) or, after 10 minutes, turn the pressure release valve on the lid to venting and release steam. Be careful as the steam is very hot. After the pressure has released completely, open the lid. 9. If the stew is watery, turn on the Sauté function and let it cook for a few more minutes with the lid off. 10. Add cilantro and can of black beans, combine well, and let cook for a few minutes.

**Per Serving**

Calories: 209 | fat: 3g | protein: 24g | carbs: 21g | sugars: 8g | fiber: 6g | sodium: 609mg

# Creamy Chicken Wild Rice Soup

**Prep time: 15 minutes | Cook time: 15 minutes | Serves 5**

| | |
|---|---|
| 2 tablespoons margarine | ½ cup yellow onion, diced |
| ¾ cup carrots, diced | ¾ cup sliced mushrooms (about 3–4 mushrooms) |
| ½ pound chicken breast, diced into 1-inch cubes | 6.2-ounce box Uncle Ben's Long |
| 2 (14-ounce) cans low-sodium chicken broth | Grain & Wild Rice Fast Cook |
| 1 cup skim milk | 1 cup evaporated skim milk |
| 2 ounces fat-free cream cheese | 2 tablespoons cornstarch |

1. Select the Sauté feature and add the margarine, onion, carrots, and mushrooms to the inner pot. Sauté for about 5 minutes until onions are translucent and soft. 2. Add the cubed chicken and seasoning packet from the Uncle Ben's box and stir to combine. 3. Add the rice and chicken broth. Select Manual, high pressure, then lock the lid and make sure the vent is set to sealing. Set the time for 5 minutes. 4. After the cooking time ends, allow it to stay on Keep Warm for 5 minutes and then quick release the pressure. 5. Remove the lid; change the setting to the Sauté function again. 6. Add the skim milk, evaporated milk, and cream cheese. Stir to melt. 7. In a small bowl, mix the cornstarch with a little bit of water to dissolve, then add to the soup to thicken.

**Per Serving**

Calories: 316 | fat: 7g | protein: 27g | carbs: 35g | sugars: 10g | fiber: 1g | sodium: 638mg

# Southwestern Bean Soup with Corn Dumplings

## Prep time: 50 minutes | Cook time: 4 to 12 hours | Serves 8

15½-ounce can red kidney beans, rinsed and drained

3 cups water

14½-ounce can Mexican-style stewed tomatoes

1 cup sliced carrots

4-ounce can chopped green chilies

1–2 teaspoons chili powder

2 cloves garlic, minced

**Sauce:**

⅓ cup flour

1 teaspoon baking powder

1 egg white, beaten

1 tablespoon oil

15½-ounce can black beans, pinto beans, or great northern beans, rinsed and drained

10-ounce package frozen whole-kernel corn, thawed

1 cup chopped onions

3 teaspoons sodium-free instant bouillon powder (any flavor)

¼ cup yellow cornmeal

Dash of pepper

2 tablespoons milk

1. Combine the 11 soup ingredients in inner pot of the Instant Pot. 2. Secure the lid and cook on the Low Slow Cook setting for 10–12 hours or high for 4–5 hours. 3. Make dumplings by mixing together flour, cornmeal, baking powder, and pepper. 4. Combine egg white, milk, and oil. Add to flour mixture. Stir with fork until just combined. 5. At the end of the soup's cooking time, turn the Instant Pot to Slow Cook function high if you don't already have it there. Remove the lid and drop dumpling mixture by rounded teaspoonfuls to make 8 mounds atop the soup. 6. Secure the lid once more and cook for an additional 30 minutes.

**Per Serving**

Calories: 197 | fat: 1g | protein: 9g | carbs: 39g | sugars: 6g | fiber: 8g | sodium: 367mg

# Golden Lentil–Pea Soup

## Prep time: 10 minutes | Cook time: 50 minutes | Serves 6

1 cup diced onion

1 tablespoon smoked paprika

1 teaspoon ground cumin

¼ teaspoon sea salt

4 cups chopped yellow sweet potato (or 2 cups chopped sweet potato and 2 cups chopped carrot)

2 cups vegetable broth

1 cup chopped celery

1 teaspoon dried rosemary

¼ teaspoon allspice

2–3 tablespoons + 4 cups water

1½ cups dried red lentils

1 cup dried yellow split peas

1½ tablespoons apple cider vinegar

1. In a large soup pot over medium-high heat, combine the onion, celery, paprika, rosemary, cumin, allspice, salt, and 2 to 3 tablespoons of the water, and stir. Cook for 8 to 9 minutes, then add the potato, lentils, split peas, broth, and the remaining 4 cups of water. Stir to combine. Increase the heat to high to bring to a boil. Reduce the heat to low, cover, and simmer for 40 to 45 minutes, or until the peas are completely softened. Stir in the apple cider vinegar, season with additional salt and pepper if desired, and serve.

**Per Serving**

Calorie: 340 | fat: 1g | protein: 21g | carbs: 64g | sugars: 8g | fiber: 20g | sodium: 363mg

# Chicken Brunswick Stew

**Prep time: 0 minutes | Cook time: 30 minutes | Serves 6**

2 tablespoons extra-virgin olive oil
1 large yellow onion, diced
1 teaspoon dried thyme
1 teaspoon smoked paprika
½ teaspoon freshly ground black pepper
1 tablespoon hot sauce (such as Tabasco or Crystal)
1½ cups frozen corn
One 14½-ounce can fire-roasted diced tomatoes and their liquid

2 garlic cloves, chopped
2 pounds boneless, skinless chicken (breasts, tenders, or thighs), cut into bite-size pieces
1 teaspoon fine sea salt
1 cup low-sodium chicken broth
1 tablespoon raw apple cider vinegar
1½ cups frozen baby lima beans
2 tablespoons tomato paste
Cornbread, for serving

1. Select the Sauté setting on the Instant Pot and heat the oil and garlic for 2 minutes, until the garlic is bubbling but not browned. Add the onion and sauté for 3 minutes, until it begins to soften. Add the chicken and sauté for 3 minutes more, until mostly opaque. The chicken does not have to be cooked through. Add the thyme, paprika, salt, and pepper and sauté for 1 minute more. 2. Stir in the broth, hot sauce, vinegar, corn, and lima beans. Add the diced tomatoes and their liquid in an even layer and dollop the tomato paste on top. Do not stir them in. 3. Secure the lid and set the Pressure Release to Sealing. Press the Cancel button to reset the cooking program, then select the Pressure Cook or Manual setting and set the cooking time for 5 minutes at high pressure. (The pot will take about 15 minutes to come up to pressure before the cooking program begins.) 4. When the cooking program ends, let the pressure release naturally for at least 10 minutes, then move the Pressure Release to Venting to release any remaining steam. Open the pot and stir the stew to mix all of the ingredients. 5. Ladle the stew into bowls and serve hot, with cornbread alongside.

**Per Serving**

Calories: 349 | fat: 7g | protein: 40g | carbs: 17g | sugars: 7g | fiber: 7g | sodium: 535mg

# Favorite Chili

**Prep time: 10 minutes | Cook time: 35 minutes | Serves 5**

1 pound extra-lean ground beef
½ teaspoons black pepper
1 small onion, chopped
1 green pepper, chopped
½ teaspoons cumin
16-ounce can chili beans

1 teaspoon salt
1 tablespoon olive oil
2 cloves garlic, minced
2 tablespoons chili powder
1 cup water
15-ounce can low-sodium crushed tomatoes

1. Press Sauté button and adjust once to Sauté More function. Wait until indicator says "hot." 2. Season the ground beef with salt and black pepper. 3. Add the olive oil into the inner pot. Coat the whole bottom of the pot with the oil. 4. Add ground beef into the inner pot. The ground beef will start to release moisture. Allow the ground beef to brown and crisp slightly, stirring occasionally to break it up. Taste and adjust the seasoning with more salt and ground black pepper. 5. Add diced onion, minced garlic, chopped pepper, chili powder, and cumin. Sauté for about 5 minutes, until the spices start to release their fragrance. Stir frequently. 6. Add water and 1 can of chili beans, not drained. Mix well. Pour in 1 can of crushed tomatoes. 7. Close and secure lid, making sure vent is set to sealing, and pressure cook on Manual at high pressure for 10 minutes. 8. Let the pressure release naturally when cooking time is up. Open the lid carefully.

**Per Serving**

Calories: 213 | fat: 10g | protein: 18g | carbs: 11g | sugars: 4g | fiber: 4g | sodium: 385mg

# Pork Chili

## Prep time: 15 minutes | Cook time: 4 hour to 8 minutes | Serves 5

1 pound boneless pork ribs
4¼-ounce cans diced green chiles, drained
1 clove garlic, minced

2 14½-ounce cans fire-roasted diced tomatoes
½ cup chopped onion
1 tablespoon chili powder

1. Layer the ingredients into the Instant Pot inner pot in the order given. 2. Secure the lid. Cook on the high Slow Cook function for 4 hours or on low 6–8 hours, or until pork is tender but not dry. 3. Cut up or shred meat. Stir into the chili and serve.

**Per Serving**
Calories: 180 | fat: 7g | protein: 18g | carbs: 12g | sugars: 6g | fiber: 3g | sodium: 495mg

# Easy Southern Brunswick Stew

## Prep time: 20 minutes | Cook time: 8 minutes | Serves 12

2 pounds pork butt, visible fat removed
1¼ cups ketchup
10-ounce package frozen peas
Hot sauce to taste, optional

17-ounce can white corn
2 cups diced, cooked potatoes
2 (10¾-ounce) cans reduced-sodium tomato soup

1. Place pork in the Instant Pot and secure the lid. 2. Press the Slow Cook setting and cook on low 6–8 hours. 3. When cook time is over, remove the meat from the bone and shred, removing and discarding all visible fat. 4. Combine all the meat and remaining ingredients (except the hot sauce) in the inner pot of the Instant Pot. 5. Secure the lid once more and cook in Slow Cook mode on low for 30 minutes more. Add hot sauce if you wish.

**Per Serving**
Calories: 213 | fat: 7g | protein: 13g | carbs: 27g | sugars: 9g | fiber: 3g | sodium: 584mg

# Instantly Good Beef Stew

## Prep time: 20 minutes | Cook time: 35 minutes | Serves 6

3 tablespoons olive oil, divided
2 cloves garlic, minced
3 ribs celery, sliced
2–3 carrots, sliced
10 ounces low-sodium beef broth
¼ teaspoon pepper

2 pounds stewing beef, cubed
1 large onion, chopped
3 large potatoes, cubed
8 ounces no-salt-added tomato sauce
2 teaspoons Worcestershire sauce
1 bay leaf

1. Set the Instant Pot to the Sauté function, then add in 1 tablespoon of the oil. Add in ⅓ of the beef cubes and brown and sear all sides. Repeat this process twice more with the remaining oil and beef cubes. Set the beef aside. 2. Place the garlic, onion, and celery into the pot and sauté for a few minutes. Press Cancel. 3. Add the beef back in as well as all of the remaining ingredients. 4. Secure the lid and make sure the vent is set to sealing. Choose Manual for 35 minutes. 5. When cook time is up, let the pressure release naturally for 15 minutes, then release any remaining pressure manually. 6. Remove the lid, remove the bay leaf, then serve.

**Per Serving**
Calories: 401 | fat: 20g | protein: 35g | carbs: 19g | sugars: 5g | fiber: 3g | sodium: 157mg

# Cauliflower Chili

## Prep time: 10 minutes | Cook time: 35 minutes | Serves 5

2 cups thickly sliced carrot

4 or 5 cloves garlic, minced

1½ cups diced onion

1½ tablespoons mild chili powder

2 teaspoons ground cumin

⅛ teaspoon allspice

1 can (28 ounces) crushed tomatoes

1 can (15 ounces) kidney beans or black beans, rinsed and drained

½ large or 1 full small head cauliflower

1 tablespoon balsamic vinegar

1 teaspoon sea salt

1 tablespoon cocoa powder

2 teaspoons dried oregano

¼ teaspoon crushed red-pepper flakes (or to taste)

1 can (15 ounces) pinto beans, rinsed and drained

½ cup water

Lime wedges

1. In a food processor, combine the carrot, cauliflower, and garlic, and pulse until finely minced. (Alternatively, you could mince by hand.) In a large pot over medium heat, combine the vinegar, onion, salt, chili powder, cocoa, cumin, oregano, allspice, and red-pepper flakes. Cook for 3 to 4 minutes, stirring occasionally. Add the minced carrot, cauliflower, and garlic, and cook for 5 to 6 minutes, stirring occasionally. Add the tomatoes, pinto and kidney beans, and water, and stir to combine. Increase the heat to high to bring to a boil. Reduce the heat to low, cover, and simmer for 25 minutes. Taste, and season as desired. Serve with lime wedges.

**Per Serving**

Calorie: 237 | fat: 3g | protein: 13g | carbs: 45g | sugars: 13g | fiber: 15g | sodium: 1036mg

# Jamaican Stew

## Prep time: 10 minutes | Cook time: 20 minutes | Serves 4

1½ cups chopped onions

1¼ teaspoons sea salt

1½ teaspoons ground coriander

½ teaspoon ground turmeric

½ teaspoon ground allspice

1 small can (5.5 ounces) light coconut milk

2 cans (15 ounces each) black beans or adzuki beans, rinsed and drained

3 tablespoons freshly squeezed lime juice

¼ cup freshly chopped cilantro (optional)

3–4 cups cubed plantains (see Note; can substitute sweet potatoes)

½ teaspoon ground cumin

1 teaspoon dried thyme

¼ teaspoon crushed red-pepper flakes (or to taste)

3½ cups water

3 cups cauliflower florets

2 tablespoons freshly grated ginger

3 cups baby spinach leaves

Lime wedges for serving

1. In a large pot over medium or medium-high heat, combine the onion, plantains, salt, coriander, cumin, turmeric, thyme, allspice, red-pepper flakes, and a few tablespoons of the coconut milk. Cook for 6 to 7 minutes, stirring occasionally. Add the water, beans, cauliflower, ginger, and remaining coconut milk. Increase the heat to high to bring to a boil, then reduce the heat to low, cover, and cook for 12 to 15 minutes, or until the plantains are cooked through. Add the lime juice, spinach, and cilantro (if using), and stir just until the spinach wilts. Serve immediately, with the lime wedges.

**Per Serving**

Calorie: 426 | fat: 5g | protein: 16g | carbs: 88g | sugars: 22g | fiber: 22g | sodium: 1053mg

# Green Chile Corn Chowder

## Prep time: 20 minutes | Cook time: 7 to 8 hours | Serves 8

16-ounce can cream-style corn
2 tablespoons chopped fresh chives
2-ounce jar chopped pimentos, drained
2 (10½-ounce cans) 100% fat-free
lower-sodium chicken broth
1 cup fat-free milk

3 potatoes, peeled and diced
4-ounce can diced green chilies, drained
½ cup chopped cooked ham
Pepper to taste
Tabasco sauce to taste

1. Combine all ingredients, except milk, in the inner pot of the Instant Pot. 2. Secure the lid and cook using the Slow Cook function on low 7–8 hours or until potatoes are tender. 3. When cook time is up, remove the lid and stir in the milk. Cover and let simmer another 20 minutes.

**Per Serving**
Calories: 124 | fat: 2g | protein: 6g | carbs: 21g | sugars: 7g | fiber: 2g | sodium: 563mg

# Savory Beef Stew with Mushrooms and Turnips

## Prep time: 0 minutes | Cook time: 55 minutes | Serves 6

1½ pounds beef stew meat
¾ teaspoon freshly ground black pepper
3 garlic cloves, minced
2 celery stalks, diced
1 cup low-sodium roasted beef bone broth
1 tablespoon Dijon mustard
1 bay leaf
8 ounces carrots, cut into 1-inch-thick rounds
1 pound parsnips, halved lengthwise,
then cut crosswise into 1-inch pieces

¾ teaspoon fine sea salt
1 tablespoon cold-pressed avocado oil
1 yellow onion, diced
8 ounces cremini mushrooms, quartered
2 tablespoons Worcestershire sauce
1 teaspoon dried rosemary, crumbled
3 tablespoons tomato paste
1 pound turnips, cut into 1-inch pieces

1. Sprinkle the beef all over with the salt and pepper. 2. Select the Sauté setting on the Instant Pot and heat the oil and garlic for 2 minutes, until the garlic is bubbling but not browned. Add the onion, celery, and mushrooms and sauté for 5 minutes, until the onion begins to soften and the mushrooms are giving up their liquid. Stir in the broth, Worcestershire sauce, mustard, rosemary, and bay leaf. Stir in the beef. Add the tomato paste in a dollop on top. Do not stir it in. 3. Secure the lid and set the Pressure Release to Sealing. Press the Cancel button to reset the cooking program, then select the Meat/Stew, Pressure Cook, or Manual setting and set the cooking time for 20 minutes at high pressure. (The pot will take about 10 minutes to come up to pressure before the cooking program begins.) 4. When the cooking program ends, perform a quick pressure release by moving the Pressure Release to Venting, or let the pressure release naturally. Open the pot, remove and discard the bay leaf, and stir in the tomato paste. Place the carrots, turnips, and parsnips on top of the meat. 5. Secure the lid and set the Pressure Release to Sealing. Press the Cancel button to reset the cooking program, then select the Pressure Cook or Manual setting and set the cooking time for 3 minutes at low pressure. (The pot will take about 15 minutes to come up to pressure before the cooking program begins.) 6. When the cooking program ends, perform a quick pressure release by moving the Pressure Release to Venting. Open the pot and stir to combine all of the ingredients. 7. Ladle the stew into bowls and serve hot.

**Per Serving**
Calories: 304 | fat: 8g | protein: 29g | carbs: 30g | sugars: 10g | fiber: 8g | sodium: 490mg

# Chicken Vegetable Soup

## Prep time: 12 to 25 minutes | Cook time: 4 minutes | Serves 6

1–2 raw chicken breasts, cubed
4 cloves garlic, minced
1 large carrot, peeled and cubed
½ cup frozen corn
¼ cup frozen lima beans
¼–½ cup chopped savoy cabbage
3 cups low-sodium chicken bone broth
1 teaspoon garlic powder
¼–½ teaspoon red pepper flakes

½ medium onion, chopped
½ sweet potato, small cubes
4 stalks celery, chopped, leaves included
¼ cup frozen peas
1 cup frozen green beans (bite-sized)
14½-ounce can low-sodium petite diced tomatoes
½ teaspoon black pepper
¼ cup chopped fresh parsley

1. Add all of the ingredients, in the order listed, to the inner pot of the Instant Pot. 2. Lock the lid in place, set the vent to sealing, press Manual, and cook at high pressure for 4 minutes. 3. Release the pressure manually as soon as cooking time is finished.
**Per Serving**
Calories: 176 | fat: 3g | protein: 21g | carbs: 18g | sugars: 7g | fiber: 4g | sodium: 169mg

# French Onion Soup

## Prep time: 10 minutes | Cook time: 20 minutes | Serves 10

½ cup light, soft tub margarine
3 14-ounce cans 98% fat-free,
lower-sodium beef broth
1½ teaspoons Worcestershire sauce
10 (1-ounce) slices French bread, toasted

8–10 large onions, sliced
2½ cups water
3 teaspoons sodium-free chicken bouillon powder
3 bay leaves

1. Turn the Instant Pot to the Sauté function and add in the margarine and onions. Cook about 5 minutes, or until the onions are slightly soft. Press Cancel. 2. Add the beef broth, water, bouillon powder, Worcestershire sauce, and bay leaves and stir. 3. Secure the lid and make sure vent is set to sealing. Cook on Manual mode for 20 minutes. 4. Let the pressure release naturally for 15 minutes, then do a quick release. Open the lid and discard bay leaves. 5. Ladle into bowls. Top each with a slice of bread and some cheese if you desire.
**Per Serving**
Calories: 178 | fat: 4g | protein: 6g | carbs: 31g | sugars: 10g | fiber: 4g | sodium: 476mg

# Italian Vegetable Soup

## Prep time: 20 minutes | Cook time: 5 to 9 hours | Serves 6

3 small carrots, sliced
2 small potatoes, diced
1 garlic clove, minced
1¼ teaspoons dried basil
16-ounce can red kidney beans, undrained
14½-ounce can stewed tomatoes, with juice

1 small onion, chopped
2 tablespoons chopped parsley
3 teaspoons sodium-free beef bouillon powder
¼ teaspoon pepper
3 cups water
1 cup diced, extra-lean, lower-sodium cooked ham

1. In the inner pot of the Instant Pot, layer the carrots, onion, potatoes, parsley, garlic, beef bouillon, basil, pepper, and kidney beans. Do not stir. Add water. 2. Secure the lid and cook on the Low Slow Cook mode for 8–9 hours, or on high 4½–5½ hours, until vegetables are tender. 3. Remove the lid and stir in the tomatoes and ham. Secure the lid again and cook on high Slow Cook mode for 10–15 minutes more.
**Per Serving**
Calories: 156 | fat: 1g | protein: 9g | carbs: 29g | sugars: 8g | fiber: 5g | sodium: 614mg

# Sweet Potato Bisque with White Beans

**Prep time: 10 minutes | Cook time: 40 minutes | Serves 4**

1½ tablespoons balsamic vinegar
1 cup chopped red pepper (roasted or raw)
1 teaspoon dried rosemary or 2 teaspoons fresh, roughly chopped
Freshly ground black pepper to taste
1½–2 teaspoons Dijon mustard
2 cans (15 ounces each) white beans, drained and rinsed

2 cups chopped onions
1¼ teaspoons sea salt + more to taste
1 teaspoon paprika (can substitute smoked paprika, for extra flavor)
3–3½ cups peeled, cubed yellow sweet potatoes
4 cups water

1. In a soup pot over medium-high heat, combine the vinegar, onions, red pepper, salt, rosemary, paprika, and black pepper. Cover, reduce the heat to medium or medium-low, and cook for 8 to 9 minutes, or until the onions are softened and starting to caramelize. Add the sweet potatoes and mustard, and stir with 1 to 2 tablespoons of the water. Cover and cook for a few minutes. Add the remaining water and increase the heat to high to bring to a boil. Reduce the heat to low, cover, and simmer for 15 to 20 minutes, or until the sweet potatoes are cooked through. Turn off the heat and add 1 cup of the white beans. Use an immersion blender to puree until the bisque is smooth and silky. Add the remaining beans, cover, and simmer for 5 to 10 minutes. Serve.

**Per Serving**
Calorie: 327 | fat: 1g | protein: 17g | carbs: 65g | sugars: 12g | fiber: 13g | sodium: 1044mg

# Black Bean, Turmeric, and Cauliflower Tortilla Soup

**Prep time: 10 minutes | Cook time: 45 minutes | Serves 4**

1 medium head cauliflower, chopped into medium florets
½ teaspoon garlic powder
1 clove garlic, minced
2 cups (480 ml) low-sodium salsa
4 cups (960 ml) water
1 (15-ounce [425-g]) can black beans, drained and rinsed
Avocado, sliced (optional)

2 teaspoons (10 ml) extra virgin olive oil, divided
½ teaspoon ground turmeric
1 medium yellow onion, coarsely chopped
1 medium red bell pepper, coarsely chopped
1 teaspoon chipotle chili powder (see Tips)
Juice of ½ medium lime
½ cup (60 g) shredded Cheddar cheese
Finely chopped fresh cilantro, as needed
4 lime wedges

1. Preheat the oven to 425°F (218°C). 2. Place the cauliflower florets in a large bowl. Add 1 teaspoon of the oil, turmeric, and garlic powder and toss the cauliflower florets to coat them in the seasonings. Transfer the cauliflower to a large baking sheet. Bake the cauliflower for 25 minutes, until it is golden brown. 3. Meanwhile, heat the remaining 1 teaspoon of oil in a large pot over medium heat. Add the onion, garlic, and bell pepper and sauté the vegetables for 5 to 10 minutes, or until the onion is translucent with charred edges. Add the salsa, chipotle chili powder, water, lime juice, and black beans and bring the soup to a simmer. 4. When the cauliflower is done, add it and the Cheddar cheese to the soup. Simmer the soup for at least 15 to 20 minutes to allow the flavors to meld. 5. Serve the soup with the cilantro sprinkled on top, avocado if desired, and a lime wedge on the side of each serving.

**Per Serving**
Calorie: 347 | fat: 7g | protein: 13g | carbs: 62g | sugars: 15g | fiber: 13g | sodium: 268mg

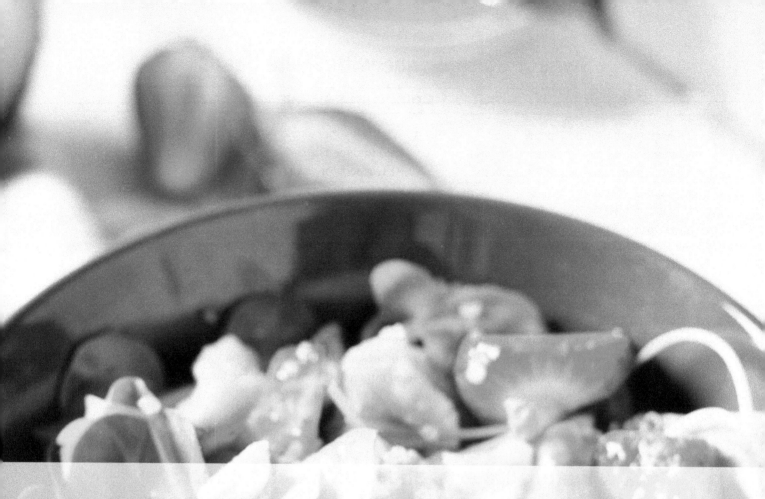

# Chapter 9   Vegetables and Sides

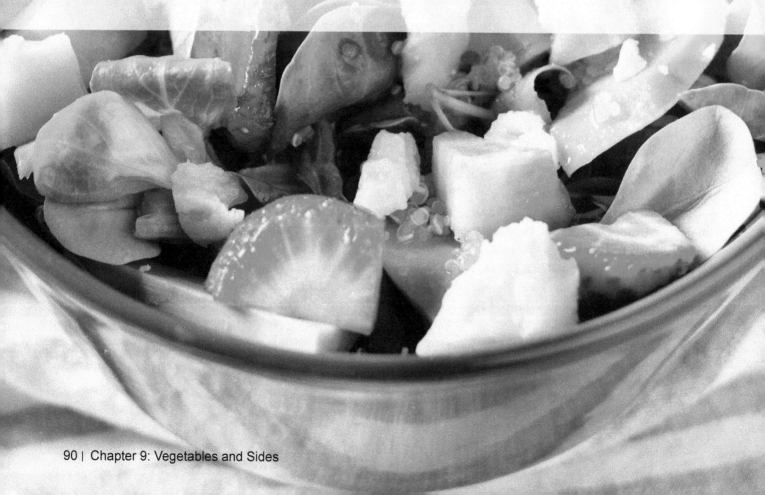

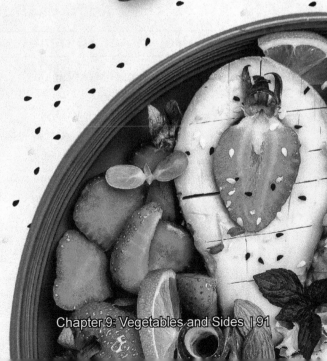

# Vegetable Medley

## Prep time: 20 minutes | Cook time: 2 minutes | Serves 8

2 medium parsnips
1 turnip, about 4½ inches diameter
1 teaspoon salt
2 tablespoons canola or olive oil

4 medium carrots
1 cup water
3 tablespoons sugar
½ teaspoon salt

1. Clean and peel vegetables. Cut in 1-inch pieces. 2. Place the cup of water and 1 teaspoon salt into the Instant Pot's inner pot with the vegetables. 3. Secure the lid and make sure vent is set to sealing. Press Manual and set for 2 minutes. 4. When cook time is up, release the pressure manually and press Cancel. Drain the water from the inner pot. 5. Press Sauté and stir in sugar, oil, and salt. Cook until sugar is dissolved. Serve.

**Per Serving**

Calories: 63 | fat: 2g | protein: 1g | carbs: 12g | sugars: 6g | fiber: 2g | sodium: 327mg

# Lean Green Avocado Mashed Potatoes

## Prep time: 15 minutes | Cook time: 30 minutes | Serves 4

2 large russet potatoes, chopped
2 medium leeks, washed and coarsely chopped
1 tablespoon dried rosemary
2 cloves garlic
2 tablespoons finely chopped fresh chives

1 large head cauliflower, cut into 1-inch (2.5-cm) florets
2 teaspoons olive oil
1 tablespoon dried thyme
1 medium avocado, peeled and pitted

1. Preheat the oven to 400°F (204°C). 2. Spread out the potatoes, cauliflower, and leeks on a large baking sheet. Drizzle the vegetables with the oil, then sprinkle them with the rosemary and thyme. Add the garlic to the baking sheet. Bake the vegetables for about 30 minutes, until the potatoes are fork-tender. 3. Transfer the vegetables to a food processor and add the avocado. Process the mixture to the desired consistency. 4. Top the mashed potatoes with the chives and serve.

**Per Serving**

Calorie: 248 | fat: 10g | protein: 7g | carbs: 37g | sugars: 6g | fiber: 9g | sodium: 69mg

# Peas with Mushrooms and Thyme

## Prep time: 10 minutes | Cook time: 10 minutes | Serves 6

2 teaspoons olive, canola or soybean oil
1 cup sliced fresh mushrooms
¼ teaspoon coarse (kosher or sea) salt
1 teaspoon chopped fresh or ¼ teaspoon dried thyme leaves

1 medium onion, diced (½ cup)
1 bag (16 ounces) frozen sweet peas
⅛ teaspoon white pepper

1. In 10-inch skillet, heat oil over medium heat. Add onion and mushrooms; cook 3 minutes, stirring occasionally. Stir in peas. Cook 3 to 5 minutes, stirring occasionally, until vegetables are tender. 2. Sprinkle with salt, pepper and thyme. Serve immediately.

**Per Serving**

Calorie: 80 | fat: 1g | protein: 4g | carbs: 11g | sugars: 4g | fiber: 2g | sodium: 150mg

# Spicy Roasted Cauliflower with Lime

## Prep time: 5 minutes | Cook time: 10 minutes | Serves 4

1 cauliflower head, broken into small florets
½ teaspoon ground chipotle chili powder
Juice of 1 lime

2 tablespoons extra-virgin olive oil
½ teaspoon salt

1. Preheat the oven to 450°F. Line a rimmed baking sheet with parchment paper. 2. In a large mixing bowl, toss the cauliflower with the olive oil, chipotle chili powder, and salt. Arrange in a single layer on the prepared baking sheet. 3. Roast for 15 minutes, flip, and continue to roast for 15 more minutes until well-browned and tender. 4. Sprinkle with the lime juice, adjust the salt as needed, and serve.

**Per Serving**

Calories: 99 | fat: 7 | protein: 3g | carbs: 8g | sugars: 3g | fiber: 3g | sodium: 284mg

# Chipotle Twice-Baked Sweet Potatoes

## Prep time: 20 minutes | Cook time: 1 hour | Serves 4

4 small sweet potatoes (about 1¾ pounds)
1 chipotle chile in adobo sauce (from 7-ounce can), finely chopped
8 teaspoons reduced-fat sour cream

¼ cup fat-free half-and-half
1 teaspoon adobo sauce (from can of chipotle chiles)
½ teaspoon salt
4 teaspoons chopped fresh cilantro

1. Heat oven to 375°F. Gently scrub potatoes but do not peel. Pierce potatoes several times with fork to allow steam to escape while potatoes bake. Bake about 45 minutes or until potatoes are tender when pierced in center with a fork. 2. When potatoes are cool enough to handle, cut lengthwise down through center of potato to within ½ inch of ends and bottom. Carefully scoop out inside, leaving thin shell. In medium bowl, mash potatoes, half-and-half, chile, adobo sauce and salt with potato masher or electric mixer on low speed until light and fluffy. 3. Increase oven temperature to 400°F. In 13x9-inch pan, place potato shells. Divide potato mixture evenly among shells. Bake uncovered 20 minutes or until potato mixture is golden brown and heated through. 4. Just before serving, top each potato with 2 teaspoons sour cream and 1 teaspoon cilantro.

**Per Serving**

Calorie: 140 | fat: 1g | protein: 3g | carbs: 27g | sugars: 9g | fiber: 4g | sodium: 400mg

# Perfect Sweet Potatoes

## Prep time: 5 minutes | Cook time: 15 minutes | Serves 4 to 6

4–6 medium sweet potatoes

1 cup of water

1. Scrub skin of sweet potatoes with a brush until clean. Pour water into inner pot of the Instant Pot. Place steamer basket in the bottom of the inner pot. Place sweet potatoes on top of steamer basket. 2. Secure the lid and turn valve to seal. 3. Select the Manual mode and set to pressure cook on high for 15 minutes. 4. Allow pressure to release naturally (about 10 minutes). 5. Once the pressure valve lowers, remove lid and serve immediately.

**Per Serving**

Calories: 112 | fat: 0g | protein: 2g | carbs: 26g | sugars: 5g | fiber: 4g | sodium: 72mg

# Classic Oven-Roasted Carrots

## Prep time: 10 minutes | Cook time: 15 minutes | Serves 4

1½ poundss (680 g) large carrots, trimmed and washed

1 tablespoon (3 g) dried rosemary

Avocado oil spray, as needed

¼ teaspoon sea salt

1. Preheat the oven to 400°F (204°C). Line a large baking sheet with parchment paper. 2. Arrange the carrots on the prepared baking sheet, making sure there is at least ½ inch (13 mm) between each of them. 3. Generously spray the carrots with the avocado oil spray, and then sprinkle them with the sea salt and rosemary. Roast the carrots for 15 minutes, or until they are fork-tender.

**Per Serving**

Calorie: 72 | fat: 1g | protein: 2g | carbs: 17g | sugars: 8g | fiber: 5g | sodium: 263mg

# Sesame Broccoli

## Prep time: 5 minutes | Cook time: 4 minutes | Serves 3

1 tablespoon tahini

1½ tablespoons tamari

1 teaspoon freshly grated ginger

4–5 cups broccoli florets

1½ tablespoons coconut nectar

1 teaspoon apple cider vinegar

¼ teaspoon garlic powder

2 teaspoons sesame seeds (raw or lightly toasted)

1. In a large bowl, whisk together the tahini, nectar, tamari, vinegar, ginger, and garlic powder. Set aside. Place a steamer basket in a large pot with 2" of water. Bring to a boil over high heat. Place the broccoli in the basket and steam for 3 to 4 minutes, or until it turns bright green and is just becoming tender. Drain and pat dry the broccoli. Add the broccoli to the marinade, and toss to coat thoroughly. Sprinkle with the sesame seeds and serve.

**Per Serving**

Calorie: 115 | fat: 4g | protein: 5g | carbs: 17g | sugars: 8g | fiber: 5g | sodium: 558mg

# Asparagus-Pepper Stir-Fry

## Prep time: 25 minutes | Cook time: 5 minutes | Serves 4

1 pound fresh asparagus spears

1 medium red, yellow or orange bell pepper, cut into ¾-inch pieces

1 tablespoon reduced-sodium soy sauce

1 teaspoon canola oil

2 cloves garlic, finely chopped

1 tablespoon orange juice

½ teaspoon ground ginger

1. Break off tough ends of asparagus as far down as stalks snap easily. Cut into 1-inch pieces. 2. In 10-inch nonstick skillet or wok, heat oil over medium heat. Add asparagus, bell pepper and garlic; cook 3 to 4 minutes or until crisp-tender, stirring constantly. 3. In small bowl, mix orange juice, soy sauce and ginger until blended; stir into asparagus mixture. Cook and stir 15 to 30 seconds or until vegetables are coated.

**Per Serving**

Calorie: 40 | fat: 1.5g | protein: 2g | carbs: 6g | sugars: 3g | fiber: 2g | sodium: 135mg

# Teriyaki Chickpeas

**Prep time: 5 minutes | Cook time: 20 to 25 minutes | Serves 7**

2 cans (15 ounces each) chickpeas, rinsed and drained
1 tablespoon pure maple syrup
½–¾ teaspoon garlic powder
½ teaspoon blackstrap molasses

1½ tablespoons tamari
1 tablespoon lemon juice
½ teaspoon ground ginger

1. Preheat the oven to 450°F. Line a baking sheet with parchment paper. 2. In a large mixing bowl, combine the chickpeas, tamari, syrup, lemon juice, garlic powder, ginger, and molasses. Toss to combine. Spread evenly on the prepared baking sheet and bake for 20 to 25 minutes, or until the marinade is absorbed. Serve warm, or refrigerate to enjoy later.

**Per Serving**

Calorie: 120 | fat: 2 | protein: 6g | carbs: 20g | sugars: 5g | fiber: 5g | sodium: 382mg

# Vegetable Curry

**Prep time: 25 minutes | Cook time: 3 minutes | Serves 10**

16-ounce package baby carrots
1 pound fresh or frozen green beans,
cut in 2-inch pieces
1–2 cloves garlic, minced
28-ounce can crushed tomatoes
1½ teaspoons chicken bouillon granules
3 tablespoons minute tapioca

3 medium potatoes, unpeeled, cubed
1 medium green pepper, chopped
1 medium onion, chopped
15-ounce can garbanzo beans, drained
3 teaspoons curry powder
1¾ cups boiling water

1. Combine carrots, potatoes, green beans, pepper, onion, garlic, garbanzo beans, crushed tomatoes, and curry powder in the Instant Pot. 2. Dissolve bouillon in boiling water, then stir in tapicoa. Pour over the contents of the Instant Pot and stir. 3. Secure the lid and make sure vent is set to sealing. Press Manual and set for 3 minutes. 4. When cook time is up, manually release the pressure.

**Per Serving**

Calories: 166 | fat: 1g | protein: 6g | carbs: 35g | sugars: 10g | fiber: 8g | sodium: 436mg

# Garlicky Cabbage and Collard Greens

**Prep time: 10 minutes | Cook time: 10 minutes | Serves 8**

2 tablespoons extra-virgin olive oil
½ small green cabbage, thinly sliced
1 tablespoon low-sodium gluten-free soy sauce or tamari

1 collard greens bunch, stemmed and thinly sliced
6 garlic cloves, minced

1. In a large skillet, heat the oil over medium-high heat. 2. Add the collards to the pan, stirring to coat with oil. Sauté for 1 to 2 minutes until the greens begin to wilt. 3. Add the cabbage and stir to coat. Cover and reduce the heat to medium low. Continue to cook for 5 to 7 minutes, stirring once or twice, until the greens are tender. 4. Add the garlic and soy sauce and stir to incorporate. Cook until just fragrant, about 30 seconds longer. Serve warm and enjoy!

**Per Serving**

Calories: 72| fat: 4g | protein: 3g | carbs: 6g | sugars: 0g | fiber: 3g | sodium: 129mg

# Caramelized Onions

**Prep time: 10 minutes | Cook time: 35 minutes | Serves 8**

4 tablespoons margarine
10-ounce can chicken, or vegetable, broth

6 large Vidalia or other sweet onions, sliced into thin half rings

1. Press Sauté on the Instant Pot. Add in the margarine and let melt. 2. Once the margarine is melted, stir in the onions and sauté for about 5 minutes. Pour in the broth and then press Cancel. 3. Secure the lid and make sure vent is set to sealing. Press Manual and set time for 20 minutes. 4. When cook time is up, release the pressure manually. Remove the lid and press Sauté. Stir the onion mixture for about 10 more minutes, allowing extra liquid to cook off.

**Per Serving**
Calorie: 123 | fat: 6g | protein: 2g | carbs: 15g | sugars: 10g | fiber: 3g | sodium: 325mg

# Teriyaki Green Beans

**Prep time: 15 minutes | Cook time: 20 minutes | Serves 4**

10 ounces (283 g) button mushrooms, thinly sliced
2 tablespoons low-sodium tamari, divided
2 cloves garlic, minced
1 cup finely chopped fresh pineapple

1 tablespoon sesame oil, divided
½ teaspoon smoked paprika
1 pound (454 g) fresh green beans, trimmed and washed

1. In a large bowl, combine the mushrooms with ½ tablespoon (8 ml) of the oil, 1½ tablespoons (23 ml) of the tamari, and the smoked paprika. Let the mushrooms rest for 10 minutes to allow them to absorb the marinade. 2. If you will be roasting the mushrooms, preheat the oven to 400°F (204°C) while the mushrooms marinate. Line a large baking sheet with parchment paper. 3. Spread out the mushrooms on the prepared baking sheet. Roast them for 20 minutes, or until they are very crispy. 4. Alternatively, if you will be stir-frying the mushrooms, heat a small skillet over medium heat. Add the mushrooms and stir-fry them for about 5 minutes, until they are tender. Note that this cooking method will yield mushrooms that are less crispy than roasting, but they will still be delicious. Meanwhile, heat the remaining ½ tablespoon (8 ml) of oil in a large skillet over medium-high heat. Add the garlic and cook it for 2 minutes, or until it is brown and fragrant. Add the green beans and pineapple. Cook the mixture for 10 minutes, until the green beans are bright green and starting to soften. Add the crispy mushrooms to the skillet. Stir to combine, then serve.

**Per Serving**
Calorie: 106 | fat: 3g | protein: 6g | carbs: 17g | sugars: 9g | fiber: 5g | sodium: 257mg

# Lemony Brussels Sprouts with Poppy Seeds

## Prep time: 10 minutes | Cook time: 2 minutes | Serves 4

1 pound (454 g) Brussels sprouts
1 cup vegetable broth or chicken bone broth
½ teaspoon kosher salt
½ medium lemon

2 tablespoons avocado oil, divided
1 tablespoon minced garlic
Freshly ground black pepper, to taste
½ tablespoon poppy seeds

1. Trim the Brussels sprouts by cutting off the stem ends and removing any loose outer leaves. Cut each in half lengthwise (through the stem). 2. Set the electric pressure cooker to the Sauté/More setting. When the pot is hot, pour in 1 tablespoon of the avocado oil. 3. Add half of the Brussels sprouts to the pot, cut-side down, and let them brown for 3 to 5 minutes without disturbing. Transfer to a bowl and add the remaining tablespoon of avocado oil and the remaining Brussels sprouts to the pot. Hit Cancel and return all of the Brussels sprouts to the pot. 4. Add the broth, garlic, salt, and a few grinds of pepper. Stir to distribute the seasonings. 5. Close and lock the lid of the pressure cooker. Set the valve to sealing. 6. Cook on high pressure for 2 minutes. 7. While the Brussels sprouts are cooking, zest the lemon, then cut it into quarters. 8. When the cooking is complete, hit Cancel and quick release the pressure. 9. Once the pin drops, unlock and remove the lid. 10. Using a slotted spoon, transfer the Brussels sprouts to a serving bowl. Toss with the lemon zest, a squeeze of lemon juice, and the poppy seeds. Serve immediately.

**Per Serving**
Calories: 125 | fat: 8g | protein: 4g | carbs: 13g | sugars: 3g | fiber: 5g | sodium: 504mg

# Herb-Roasted Root Vegetables

## Prep time: 15 minutes | Cook time: 45 to 55 minutes | Serves 6

2 medium turnips, peeled, cut into
1-inch pieces (3 cups)
1 medium red onion, cut into 1-inch wedges (1 cup)
Cooking spray
½ teaspoon coarse salt

2 medium parsnips, peeled, cut into
½-inch pieces (1½ cups)
1 cup ready-to-eat baby-cut carrots
2 teaspoons Italian seasoning

1. Heat oven to 425°F. Spray 15x10x1-inch pan with cooking spray. Arrange vegetables in single layer in pan. Spray with cooking spray (2 or 3 seconds). Sprinkle with Italian seasoning and salt. 2. Bake uncovered 45 to 55 minutes, stirring once, until vegetables are tender.

**Per Serving**
Calorie: 70 | fat: 0g | protein: 1g | carbs: 15g | sugars: 7g | fiber: 4g | sodium: 260mg

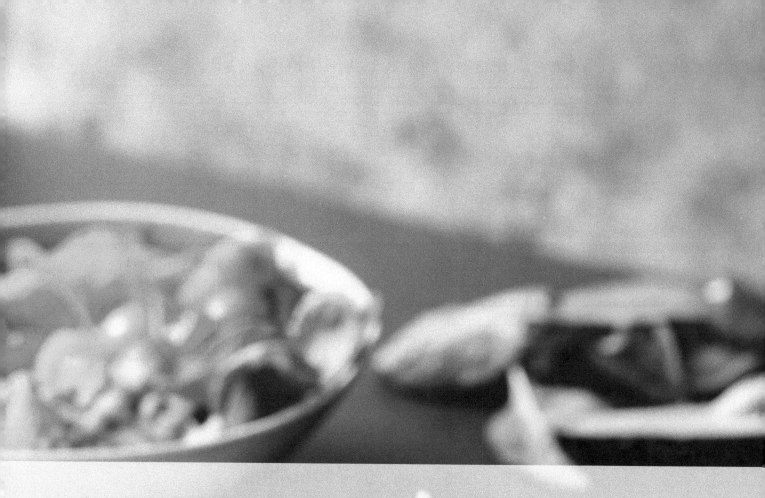

# Chapter 10   Vegetarian Mains

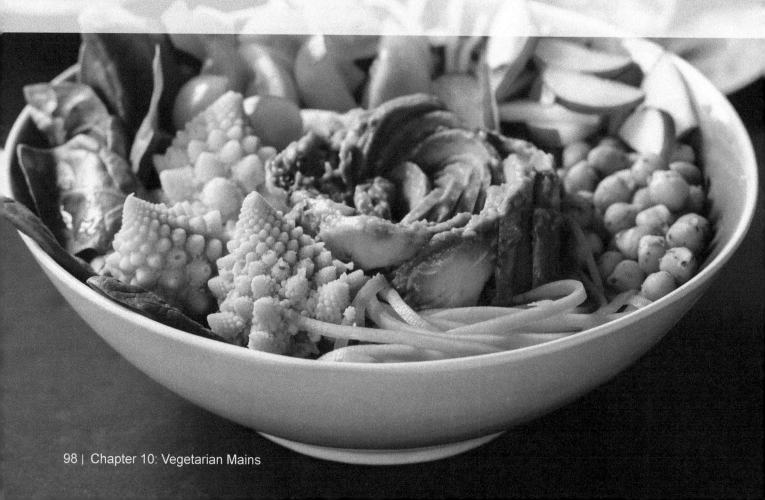

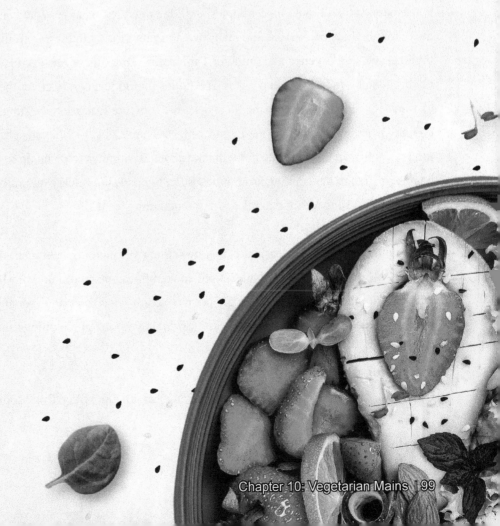

# Instant Pot Hoppin' John with Skillet Cauli "Rice"

## Prep time: 0 minutes | Cook time: 30 minutes | Serves 6

| | |
|---|---|
| Hoppin' John | 1 pound dried black-eyed peas (about 2¼ cups) |
| 8⅔ cups water | 1½ teaspoons fine sea salt |
| 2 tablespoons extra-virgin olive oil | 2 garlic cloves, minced |
| 8 ounces shiitake mushrooms, stemmed and chopped, or cremini mushrooms, chopped | 1 small yellow onion, diced |
| | 1 green bell pepper, seeded and diced |
| 2 celery stalks, diced | 2 jalapeño chiles, seeded and diced |
| ½ teaspoon smoked paprika | ½ teaspoon dried thyme |
| ½ teaspoon dried sage | ¼ teaspoon cayenne pepper |
| 2 cups low-sodium vegetable broth | Cauli "Rice" |
| 1 tablespoon vegan buttery spread or unsalted butter | 1 pound riced cauliflower |
| ½ teaspoon fine sea salt | 2 green onions, white and green parts, sliced |
| Hot sauce (such as Tabasco or Crystal) for serving | |

### Make the Hoppin' John:

1. In a large bowl, combine the black-eyed peas, 8 cups of the water, and 1 teaspoon of the salt and stir to dissolve the salt. Let soak for at least 8 hours or up to overnight. 2. Select the Sauté setting on the Instant Pot and heat the oil and garlic for 3 minutes, until the garlic is bubbling but not browned. Add the mushrooms and the remaining ½ teaspoon salt and sauté for 5 minutes, until the mushrooms have wilted and begun to give up their liquid. Add the onion, bell pepper, celery, and jalapeños and sauté for 4 minutes, until the onion is softened. Add the paprika, thyme, sage, and cayenne and sauté for 1 minute. 3. Drain the black-eyed peas and add them to the pot along with the broth and remaining ⅔ cup water. The liquid should just barely cover the beans. (Add an additional splash of water if needed.) 4. Secure the lid and set the Pressure Release to Sealing. Press the Cancel button to reset the cooking program, then select the Bean/Chili, Pressure Cook, or Manual setting and set the cooking time for 5 minutes at high pressure. (The pot will take about 10 minutes to come up to pressure before the cooking program begins.) 5. When the cooking program ends, let the pressure release naturally for 10 minutes, then move the Pressure Release to Venting to release any remaining steam.

### Make the cauli "rice":

1. While the pressure is releasing, in a large skillet over medium heat, melt the buttery spread. Add the cauliflower and salt and sauté for 3 to 5 minutes, until cooked through and piping hot. (If using frozen riced cauliflower, this may take another 2 minutes or so.) 2. Spoon the cauli "rice" onto individual plates. Open the pot and spoon the black-eyed peas on top of the cauli "rice". Sprinkle with the green onions and serve right away, with the hot sauce on the side.

### Per Serving

Calories: 287 | fat: 7g | protein: 23g | carbs: 56g | sugars: 8g | fiber: 24g | sodium: 894mg

# Pra Ram Vegetables and Peanut Sauce with Seared Tofu

## Prep time: 5 minutes | Cook time: 20 minutes | Serves 4

Peanut Sauce

2 garlic cloves, minced

½ cup coconut milk

1 tablespoon plus 1 teaspoon soy sauce,
 tamari, or coconut aminos

2 carrots, sliced on the diagonal ¼ inch thick

1 pound broccoli florets

wedges (with core intact so wedges hold together)

One 14-ounce package extra-firm tofu, drained

¼ teaspoon freshly ground black pepper

2 tablespoons coconut oil

2 tablespoons cold-pressed avocado oil

½ cup creamy natural peanut butter

2 tablespoons brown rice syrup

¼ cup water

Vegetables

8 ounces zucchini, julienned ¼ inch thick

½ small head green cabbage, cut into 1-inch-thick

Tofu

¼ teaspoon fine sea salt

1 tablespoon cornstarch

**Make the peanut sauce:**

In a small saucepan over medium heat, warm the oil and garlic for about 2 minutes, until the garlic is bubbling but not browned. Add the peanut butter, coconut milk, brown rice syrup, soy sauce, and water; stir to combine; and bring to a simmer (this will take about 3 minutes). As soon as the mixture is fully combined and at a simmer, remove from the heat and keep warm. The peanut sauce will keep in an airtight container in the refrigerator for up to 5 days.

**Make the vegetables:**

Pour 1 cup water into the Instant Pot and place a steamer basket into the pot. In order, layer the carrots, zucchini, broccoli, and cabbage in the steamer basket, finishing with the cabbage. 2. Secure the lid and set the Pressure Release to Sealing. Select the Steam setting and set the cooking time for 0 (zero) minutes at low pressure. (The pot will take about 15 minutes to come up to pressure before the cooking program begins.)

**Prepare the tofuo :**

1. While the vegetables are steaming, cut the tofu crosswise into eight ½-inch-thick slices. Cut each of the slices in half crosswise, creating squares. Sandwich the squares between double layers of paper towels or a folded kitchen towel and press firmly to wick away as much moisture as possible. Sprinkle the tofu squares on both sides with the salt and pepper, then sprinkle them on both sides with the cornstarch. Using your fingers, spread the cornstarch on the top and bottom of each square to coat evenly. 2. In a large nonstick skillet over medium-high heat, warm the oil for about 3 minutes, until shimmering. Add the tofu and sear, turning once, for about 6 minutes per side, until crispy and golden. Divide the tofu evenly among four plates. 3. When the cooking program ends, perform a quick pressure release by moving the Pressure Release to Venting. Open the pot and, wearing heat-resistant mitts, grasp the handles of the steamer basket and lift it out of the pot. 4. Divide the vegetables among the plates, arranging them around the tofu. Spoon the peanut sauce over the tofu and serve.

**Per Serving**

Calories: 380 | fat: 22g | protein: 18g | carbs: 30g | sugars: 9g | fiber: 10g | sodium: 381mg

# Vegan Dal Makhani

## Prep time: 0 minutes | Cook time: 55 minutes | Serves 6

1 cup dried kidney beans
4 cups water
1 tablespoon cold-pressed avocado oil
1-inch piece fresh ginger, peeled and minced
1 large yellow onion, diced
1 green bell pepper, seeded and diced
1 teaspoon ground turmeric
One 15-ounce can fire-roasted diced tomatoes and liquid
2 tablespoons chopped fresh cilantro

⅓ cup urad dal or beluga or Puy lentils
1 teaspoon fine sea salt
1 tablespoon cumin seeds
4 garlic cloves, minced
2 jalapeño chiles, seeded and diced
1 tablespoon garam masala
¼ teaspoon cayenne pepper (optional)
2 tablespoons vegan buttery spread
Cooked cauliflower "rice" for serving
6 tablespoons plain coconut yogurt

1. In a medium bowl, combine the kidney beans, urad dal, water, and salt and stir to dissolve the salt. Let soak for 12 hours. 2. Select the Sauté setting on the Instant Pot and heat the oil and cumin seeds for 3 minutes, until the seeds are bubbling, lightly toasted, and aromatic. Add the ginger and garlic and sauté for 1 minute, until bubbling and fragrant. Add the onion, jalapeños, and bell pepper and sauté for 5 minutes, until the onion begins to soften. 3. Add the garam masala, turmeric, cayenne (if using), and the soaked beans and their liquid and stir to mix. Pour the tomatoes and their liquid on top. Do not stir them in. 4. Secure the lid and set the Pressure Release to Sealing. Press the Cancel button to reset the cooking program, then select the Pressure Cook or Manual setting and set the cooking time for 30 minutes at high pressure. (The pot will take about 15 minutes to come up to pressure before the cooking program begins.) 5. When the cooking program ends, let the pressure release naturally for 30 minutes, then move the Pressure Release to Venting to release any remaining steam. Open the pot and stir to combine, then stir in the buttery spread. If you prefer a smoother texture, ladle 1½ cups of the dal into a blender and blend until smooth, about 30 seconds, then stir the blended mixture into the rest of the dal in the pot. 6. Spoon the cauliflower "rice" into bowls and ladle the dal on top. Sprinkle with the cilantro, top with a dollop of coconut yogurt, and serve.

**Per Serving**
Calorie: 245 | fat: 7g | protein: 11g | carbs: 37g | sugars: 4g | fiber: 10g | sodium: 518mg

# Orange Tofu

## Prep time: 10 minutes | Cook time: 20 minutes | Serves 4

⅓ cup freshly squeezed orange juice (zest orange first; see orange zest ingredient below)
½ tablespoon coconut nectar or pure maple syrup
½ tablespoon freshly grated ginger
½–1 teaspoon orange zest
Few pinches of crushed red-pepper flakes (optional)

1 tablespoon tamari
1 tablespoon tahini
2 tablespoons apple cider vinegar
1 large clove garlic, grated
¼ teaspoon sea salt
1 package (12 ounces) extra-firm tofu, sliced into ¼"–½" thick squares and patted to remove excess moisture

1. Preheat the oven to 400°F. 2. In a small bowl, combine the orange juice, tamari, tahini, nectar or syrup, vinegar, ginger, garlic, orange zest, salt, and red-pepper flakes (if using). Whisk until well combined. Pour the sauce into an 8" x 12" baking dish. Add the tofu and turn to coat both sides. Bake for 20 minutes. Add salt to taste.

**Per Serving**
Calorie: 122 | fat: 7g | protein: 10g | carbs: 7g | sugars: 4g | fiber: 1g | sodium: 410mg

# No-Bake Spaghetti Squash Casserole

**Prep time: 10 minutes | Cook time: 45 minutes | Serves 6**

**Marinara**

3 tablespoons extra-virgin olive oil

One 28-ounce can whole San Marzano tomatoes and their liquid

½ teaspoon red pepper flakes (optional)

3 garlic cloves, minced

2 teaspoons Italian seasoning

1 teaspoon fine sea salt

**Vegan Parmesan**

½ cup raw whole cashews

½ teaspoon garlic powder

2 tablespoons nutritional yeast

½ teaspoon fine sea salt

**Vegan Ricotta**

One 14-ounce package firm tofu, drained

3 tablespoons nutritional yeast

2 tablespoons extra-virgin olive oil

½ cup firmly packed fresh flat-leaf parsley leaves

1½ teaspoons Italian seasoning

1 teaspoon fine sea salt

One 3½-pound steamed spaghetti squash

½ cup raw whole cashews, soaked in water to cover for 1 to 2 hours and then drained

1 teaspoon finely grated lemon zest, plus 2 tablespoons fresh lemon juice

1 teaspoon garlic powder

½ teaspoon freshly ground black pepper

2 tablespoons chopped fresh flat-leaf parsley

**Make the marinara:**

Select the Sauté setting on the Instant Pot and heat the oil and garlic for about 2 minutes, until the garlic is bubbling but not browned. Add the tomatoes and their liquid and use a wooden spoon or spatula to crush the tomatoes against the side of the pot. Stir in the Italian seasoning, salt, and pepper flakes (if using) and cook, stirring occasionally, for about 10 minutes, until the sauce has thickened a bit. Press the Cancel button to turn off the pot and let the sauce cook from the residual heat for about 5 minutes more, until it is no longer simmering. Wearing heat-resistant mitts, lift the pot out of the housing, pour the sauce into a medium heatproof bowl, and set aside. (You can make the sauce up to 4 days in advance, then let it cool, transfer it to an airtight container, and refrigerate.)

**Make the vegan Parmesan:**

In a food processor, combine the cashews, nutritional yeast, garlic powder, and salt. Using 1-second pulses, pulse about ten times, until the mixture resembles grated Parmesan cheese. Transfer to a small bowl and set aside. Do not wash the food processor bowl and blade.

**Make the vegan ricotta:**

1. Cut the tofu crosswise into eight ½-inch-thick slices. Sandwich the slices between double layers of paper towels or a folded kitchen towel and press gently to remove excess moisture. Add the tofu to the food processor along with the cashews, nutritional yeast, oil, lemon zest, lemon juice, parsley, Italian seasoning, garlic powder, salt, and pepper. Process for about 1 minute, until the mixture is mostly smooth with flecks of parsley throughout. Set aside. 2. Return the marinara to the pot. Select the Sauté setting and heat the marinara sauce for about 3 minutes, until it starts to simmer. Add the spaghetti squash and vegan ricotta to the pot and stir to combine. Continue to heat, stirring often, for 8 to 10 minutes, until piping hot. Press the Cancel button to turn off the pot. 3. Spoon the spaghetti squash into bowls, top with the vegan Parmesan and parsley, and serve right away.

**Per Serving**

Calorie: 307 | fat: 17g | protein: 16g | carbs: 25g | sugars: 2g | fiber: 5g | sodium: 985mg

# Chile Relleno Casserole with Salsa Salad

**Prep time: 10 minutes | Cook time: 55 minutes | Serves 4**

**Casserole**

½ cup gluten-free flour (such as King Arthur or Cup4Cup brand)

½ cup nondairy milk or whole milk

1 cup nondairy cheese shreds or shredded mozzarella cheese

1 teaspoon baking powder

6 large eggs

Three 4-ounce cans fire-roasted diced green chiles, drained

**Salad**

1 head green leaf lettuce, shredded

1 green bell pepper, seeded and diced

1 jalapeño chile, seeded and diced (optional)

4 teaspoons extra-virgin olive oil

⅛ teaspoon fine sea salt

2 Roma tomatoes, seeded and diced

½ small yellow onion, diced

2 tablespoons chopped fresh cilantro

4 teaspoons fresh lime juice

**Make the casserole:**

Pour 1 cup water into the Instant Pot. Butter a 7-cup round heatproof glass dish or coat with nonstick cooking spray and place the dish on a long-handled silicone steam rack. (If you don't have the long-handled rack, use the wire metal steam rack and a homemade sling) 2. In a medium bowl, whisk together the flour and baking powder. Add the eggs and milk and whisk until well blended, forming a batter. Stir in the chiles and ¾ cup of the cheese. 3. Pour the batter into the prepared dish and cover tightly with aluminum foil. Holding the handles of the steam rack, lower the dish into the Instant Pot. 4. Secure the lid and set the Pressure Release to Sealing. Select the Pressure Cook or Manual setting and set the cooking time for 40 minutes at high pressure. (The pot will take about 10 minutes to come up to pressure before the cooking program begins.) 5. When the cooking program ends, let the pressure release naturally for at least 10 minutes, then move the Pressure Release to Venting to release any remaining steam. Open the pot and, wearing heat-resistant mitts, grasp the handles of the steam rack and lift it out of the pot. Uncover the dish, taking care not to get burned by the steam or to drip condensation onto the casserole. While the casserole is still piping hot, sprinkle the remaining ¼ cup cheese evenly on top. Let the cheese melt for 5 minutes.

**Make the salad:**

1. While the cheese is melting, in a large bowl, combine the lettuce, tomatoes, bell pepper, onion, jalapeño (if using), cilantro, oil, lime juice, and salt. Toss until evenly combined. 2. Cut the casserole into wedges. Serve warm, with the salad on the side.

**Per Serving**

Calorie: 361 | fat: 22g | protein: 21g | carbs: 23g | sugars: 8g | fiber: 3g | sodium: 421mg

# Spinach Salad with Eggs, Tempeh Bacon, and Strawberries

**Prep time: 10 minutes | Cook time: 15 minutes | Serves 4**

2 tablespoons soy sauce, tamari, or coconut aminos

1 tablespoon pure maple syrup

Freshly ground black pepper

8 large eggs

3 tablespoons extra-virgin olive oil

1 tablespoon red wine vinegar

1 teaspoon Dijon mustard

One 6-ounce bag baby spinach

12 fresh strawberries, sliced

1 tablespoon raw apple cider vinegar

½ teaspoon smoked paprika

One 8-ounce package tempeh, cut crosswise into ⅛-inch-thick slices

1 shallot, minced

1 tablespoon balsamic vinegar

¼ teaspoon fine sea salt

2 hearts romaine lettuce, torn into bite-size pieces

1. In a 1-quart ziplock plastic bag, combine the soy sauce, cider vinegar, maple syrup, paprika, and ½ teaspoon pepper and carefully agitate the bag to mix the ingredients to make a marinade. Add the tempeh, seal the bag, and turn the bag back and forth several times to coat the tempeh evenly with the marinade. Marinate in the refrigerator for at least 2 hours or up to 24 hours. 2. Pour 1 cup water into the Instant Pot and place the wire metal steam rack, an egg rack, or a steamer basket into the pot. Gently place the eggs on top of the rack or in the basket, taking care not to crack them. 3. Secure the lid and set the Pressure Release to Sealing. Select the Steam setting and set the cooking time for 3 minutes at high pressure. (The pot will take about 5 minutes to come up to pressure before the cooking program begins.) 4. While the eggs are cooking, prepare an ice bath. 5. When the cooking program ends, perform a quick pressure release by moving the Pressure Release to Venting. Open the pot and, using tongs, transfer the eggs to the ice bath to cool. 6. Remove the tempeh from the marinade and blot dry between layers of paper towels. Discard the marinade. In a large nonstick skillet over medium-high heat, warm 1 tablespoon of the oil for 2 minutes. Add the tempeh in a single layer and fry, turning once, for 2 to 3 minutes per side, until well browned. Transfer the tempeh to a plate and set aside. 7. Wipe out the skillet and set it over medium heat. Add the remaining 2 tablespoons oil and the shallot and sauté for about 2 minutes, until the shallot is golden brown. Turn off the heat and stir in the red wine vinegar, balsamic vinegar, mustard, salt, and ¼ teaspoon pepper to make a vinaigrette. 8. In a large bowl, combine the spinach and romaine. Pour in the vinaigrette and toss until all of the leaves are lightly coated. Divide the dressed greens evenly among four large serving plates or shallow bowls and arrange the strawberries and fried tempeh on top. Peel the eggs, cut them in half lengthwise, and place them on top of the salads. Top with a couple grinds of pepper and serve right away.

**Per Serving**
Calorie: 435 | fat: 25g | protein: 29g | carbs: 25g | sugars: 10g | fiber: 5g | sodium: 332mg

# Veggie Fajitas

## Prep time: 10 minutes | Cook time: 15 minutes | Serves 4

**For the guacamole**

| | |
|---|---|
| 2 small avocados pitted and peeled | 1 teaspoon freshly squeezed lime juice |
| ¼ teaspoon salt | 9 cherry tomatoes, halved |

**For the fajitas**

| | |
|---|---|
| 1 red bell pepper | 1 green bell pepper |
| 1 small white onion | Avocado oil cooking spray |
| 1 cup canned low-sodium black beans, drained and rinsed | ½ teaspoon ground cumin |
| | ¼ teaspoon chili powder |
| ¼ teaspoon garlic powder | 4 (6-inch) yellow corn tortillas |

**Make the guacamole:**
1. In a medium bowl, use a fork to mash the avocados with the lime juice and salt. 2. Gently stir in the cherry tomatoes.

**Make the fajitas:**
1. Cut the red bell pepper, green bell pepper, and onion into ½-inch slices. 2. Heat a large skillet over medium heat. When hot, coat the cooking surface with cooking spray. Put the peppers, onion, and beans into the skillet. 3. Add the cumin, chili powder, and garlic powder, and stir. 4. Cover and cook for 15 minutes, stirring halfway through. 5. Divide the fajita mixture equally between the tortillas, and top with guacamole and any preferred garnishes.

**Per Serving**
Calories: 269 | fat: 15g | protein: 8g | carbs: 30g | sugars: 5g | fiber: 11g | sodium: 175mg

# Southwest Tofu

## Prep time: 10 minutes | Cook time: 20 minutes | Serves 4

3½ tablespoons freshly squeezed lime juice
1½ teaspoons ground cumin
1 teaspoon chili powder
½ teaspoon sea salt
1 package (12 ounces) extra-firm tofu, sliced into
¼"–½" thick squares and patted to remove excess moisture

2 teaspoons pure maple syrup
1 teaspoon dried oregano leaves
½ teaspoon paprika
⅛ teaspoon allspice

1. In a 9" x 12" baking dish, combine the lime juice, syrup, cumin, oregano, chili powder, paprika, salt, and allspice. Add the tofu and turn to coat both sides. Bake uncovered for 20 minutes, or until the marinade is absorbed, turning once.

**Per Serving**
Calorie: 78 | fat: 4g | protein: 7g | carbs: 6g | sugars: 3g | fiber: 1g | sodium: 324mg

# Palak Tofu

## Prep time: 5 minutes | Cook time: 40 minutes | Serves 4

One 14-ounce package extra-firm tofu, drained
1 yellow onion, diced
3 garlic cloves, minced
½ teaspoon freshly ground black pepper
One 16-ounce bag frozen chopped spinach
One 14½-ounce can fire-roasted diced tomatoes
and their liquid
Cooked brown rice or cauliflower "rice"
or whole-grain flatbread for serving

5 tablespoons cold-pressed avocado oil
1-inch piece fresh ginger, peeled and minced
1 teaspoon fine sea salt
¼ teaspoon cayenne pepper
⅓ cup water
¼ cup coconut milk
2 teaspoons garam masala

1. Cut the tofu crosswise into eight ½-inch-thick slices. Sandwich the slices between double layers of paper towels or a folded kitchen towel and press firmly to wick away as much moisture as possible. Cut the slices into ½-inch cubes. 2. Select the Sauté setting on the Instant Pot and and heat 4 tablespoons of the oil for 2 minutes. Add the onion and sauté for about 10 minutes, until it begins to brown. 3. While the onion is cooking in the Instant Pot, in a large nonstick skillet over medium-high heat, warm the remaining 1 tablespoon oil. Add the tofu in a single layer and cook without stirring for about 3 minutes, until lightly browned. 4. Using a spatula, turn the cubes over and cook for about 3 minutes more, until browned on the other side. Remove from the heat and set aside. 5. Add the ginger and garlic to the onion in the Instant Pot and sauté for about 2 minutes, until the garlic is bubbling but not browned. Add the sautéed tofu, salt, black pepper, and cayenne and stir gently to combine, taking care not to break up the tofu. Add the spinach and stir gently. Pour in the water and then pour the tomatoes and their liquid over the top in an even layer. Do not stir them in. 6. Secure the lid and set the Pressure Release to Sealing. Press the Cancel button to reset the cooking program, then select the Manual or Pressure Cook setting and set the cooking time for 10 minutes at low pressure. (The pot will take about 15 minutes to come up to pressure before the cooking program begins.) 7. When the cooking program ends, let the pressure release naturally for 10 minutes, then move the Pressure Release to Venting to release any remaining steam. Open the pot, add the coconut milk and garam masala, and stir to combine. 8. Ladle the tofu onto plates or into bowls. Serve piping hot, with the "rice" alongside.

**Per Serving**
Calories: 345 | fat: 24g | protein: 14g | carbs: 18g | sugars: 5g | fiber: 6g | sodium: 777mg

# Appendix 1 Measurement Conversion Chart

## VOLUME EQUIVALENTS(DRY)

| US STANDARD | METRIC (APPROXIMATE) |
|---|---|
| 1/8 teaspoon | 0.5 mL |
| 1/4 teaspoon | 1 mL |
| 1/2 teaspoon | 2 mL |
| 3/4 teaspoon | 4 mL |
| 1 teaspoon | 5 mL |
| 1 tablespoon | 15 mL |
| 1/4 cup | 59 mL |
| 1/2 cup | 118 mL |
| 3/4 cup | 177 mL |
| 1 cup | 235 mL |
| 2 cups | 475 mL |
| 3 cups | 700 mL |
| 4 cups | 1 L |

## WEIGHT EQUIVALENTS

| US STANDARD | METRIC (APPROXIMATE) |
|---|---|
| 1 ounce | 28 g |
| 2 ounces | 57 g |
| 5 ounces | 142 g |
| 10 ounces | 284 g |
| 15 ounces | 425 g |
| 16 ounces (1 pound) | 455 g |
| 1.5 pounds | 680 g |
| 2 pounds | 907 g |

## VOLUME EQUIVALENTS(LIQUID)

| US STANDARD | US STANDARD (OUNCES) | METRIC (APPROXIMATE) |
|---|---|---|
| 2 tablespoons | 1 fl.oz. | 30 mL |
| 1/4 cup | 2 fl.oz. | 60 mL |
| 1/2 cup | 4 fl.oz. | 120 mL |
| 1 cup | 8 fl.oz. | 240 mL |
| 1 1/2 cup | 12 fl.oz. | 355 mL |
| 2 cups or 1 pint | 16 fl.oz. | 475 mL |
| 4 cups or 1 quart | 32 fl.oz. | 1 L |
| 1 gallon | 128 fl.oz. | 4 L |

## TEMPERATURES EQUIVALENTS

| FAHRENHEIT(F) | CELSIUS(C) (APPROXIMATE) |
|---|---|
| 225 °F | 107 °C |
| 250 °F | 120 °C |
| 275 °F | 135 °C |
| 300 °F | 150 °C |
| 325 °F | 160 °C |
| 350 °F | 180 °C |
| 375 °F | 190 °C |
| 400 °F | 205 °C |
| 425 °F | 220 °C |
| 450 °F | 235 °C |
| 475 °F | 245 °C |
| 500 °F | 260 °C |

# Appendix 2 The Dirty Dozen and Clean Fifteen

The Environmental Working Group (EWG) is a nonprofit, nonpartisan organization dedicated to protecting human health and the environment Its mission is to empower people to live healthier lives in a healthier environment. This organization publishes an annual list of the twelve kinds of produce, in sequence, that have the highest amount of pesticide residue-the Dirty Dozen-as well as a list of the fifteen kinds ofproduce that have the least amount of pesticide residue-the Clean Fifteen.

## THE DIRTY DOZEN

- The 2016 Dirty Dozen includes the following produce. These are considered among the year's most important produce to buy organic:

| | |
|---|---|
| Strawberries | Spinach |
| Apples | Tomatoes |
| Nectarines | Bell peppers |
| Peaches | Cherry tomatoes |
| Celery | Cucumbers |
| Grapes | Kale/collard greens |
| Cherries | Hot peppers |

- *The Dirty Dozen list contains two additional itemskale/collard greens and hot peppers-because they tend to contain trace levels of highly hazardous pesticides.*

## THE CLEAN FIFTEEN

- The least critical to buy organically are the Clean Fifteen list. The following are on the 2016 list:

| | |
|---|---|
| Avocados | Papayas |
| Corn | Kiw |
| Pineapples | Eggplant |
| Cabbage | Honeydew |
| Sweet peas | Grapefruit |
| Onions | Cantaloupe |
| Asparagus | Cauliflower |
| Mangos | |

- *Some of the sweet corn sold in the United States are made from genetically engineered (GE) seedstock. Buy organic varieties of these crops to avoid GE produce.*